Praise for
Fit *for the* King

"That a Christian's life should include service to others is an undisputed fact. But as Dr. John Madeira knows and explores in his book, Fit for the King, this cannot happen unless we first serve ourselves — unless we accept responsibility for living the healthiest lives possible so we are able to do the good works and fight the tough battles our Lord intends us to. Honor yourself by reading this book and position yourself to play a larger role as a true servant of God here on Earth."

SIMON T. BAILEY
Author of *Release Your Brilliance*
Windermere, FL

"As a personal friend and physician to our family, Dr. John has done far more than minister wise medical care to us. He really cares! This book was born out of his deep desire to see people live healthy lives and his insights will help you to enjoy optimal health. It's time for Christians to walk in the divine health that God intended. Alert. Empowered. Released to become all that we are in Christ. Let's join Dr. John on this exciting journey toward physical, emotional and spiritual fitness. Not simply fitness for fitness' sake but toward the lofty goal of becoming Fit for the King!"

DAVE HESS
Senior Pastor, Christ Com~~~~~~~ ~~~~~~ C~~~ Hill, PA
Author of *H~*

"Many 'experts' proffer life-altering truths but you can't get beyond their smugness and self-promotion. Not so with Dr. John Madeira. He offers exigent life-altering wisdom without the hyperbole. Please don't read Fit for the King if you're looking for trite, worn-out wellness platitudes. Read it to change your health and your life."

W. GREGORY LARSH, PH.D.
Senior Pastor, Windsor Chapel
Princeton, NJ

"The principles in this book are a blueprint for vibrant, abundant health. Put them into action in your daily life and experience the joy and satisfaction of impacting and increasing the kingdom of God."

DR. ROBERT DEMARIA
Drugless Healthcare Solutions
Author of the "Dr. Bob" Guide Series

"A deeply meaningful, life-changing book. You will be instructed and inspired by these truths. Dr. John has helped me realize that to be an effective pastor and Christian I need to be Fit for the King.*"*

REVEREND AL FRANK
Senior Pastor, Conoy Brethren in Christ Church,
Elizabethtown, PA

"As a pastor for almost 40 years, I've had the privilege of ministering to many people. My heart goes out to those who are struggling and suffering from so many health concerns. In Hosea 4:6 God's word says, "My people are destroyed for lack of knowledge.

In Fit for the King Dr. John provides the wisdom and counsel that Christians desperately need to claim the divine health God desires for his people. Dr. John is a sincere Christian whose daily life blesses and motivates both his patients and friends.

I have read many personal fitness and health books in my lifetime, but Fit for the King offers the most balanced approach I have ever encountered. Read it to discover the truth of God's word concerning your health and become a good steward of your body for His glory!"

―――✥―――

MEL WEAVER

Senior Pastor, Grace Chapel
Elizabethtown, PA

"Walking in divine health is the only way to fully experience your God-given destiny and avoid devastating suffering and disease. Dr. John Madeira is an expert in his field and graciously shares his wealth of knowledge. He communicates his message in a unique but practical way, providing information and revelation which will help you enjoy a long, healthy life. Fit for the King is a must read for every Christian who is serious about accomplishing all God has called them to do for the kingdom."

―――✥―――

DR. STEVE BALL

Metro Tabernacle, Pastor, Entrepreneur, Author, Motivational Speaker,
Chattanooga, TN

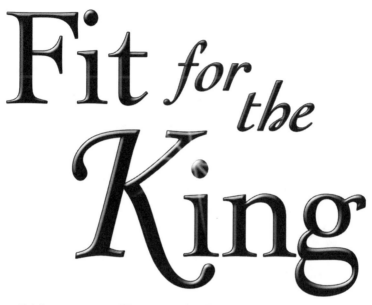

Fit for the King

WALK IN DIVINE HEALTH
EVERY DAY OF YOUR LIFE

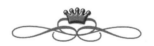

DR. JOHN MADEIRA

Fit *for the* King:
Walk in Divine Health Every Day of Your Life

ISBN: 978-0-578-02369-4

Printed in the United States of America

Maddog Publishing
158 West Caracas Avenue
Hershey, PA 17033
717-533-4840
joyce@madeirasuccess.com

Cover and Interior Book Design: Peri Poloni-Gabriel,
Knockout Design, www.knockoutbooks.com

Disclaimer

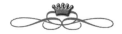

THE INFORMATION CONTAINED IN THIS BOOK
is the culmination of nearly thirty years of experience in
natural health care working directly with literally thousands of
patients of all ages in a clinical setting. The opinions expressed
are the opinions of the author and most, but not all, are sup-
ported by research. Your results will vary. The statements made
have not been evaluated by the FDA. Neither the author nor the
publisher of this material shall have liability or responsibility
to any person or entity with respect to any loss, damage, or
injury caused or alleged to be caused directly or indirectly by the
information contained in this book. The information contained
herein is not intended to be a substitute for medical counseling. It is for informational purposes only and is not intended
to diagnose, treat, or cure disease or to take the place of care
or treatment by a qualified, licensed health care professional.
Do not alter your medication, start any exercise program or
diet without first consulting your personal physician or other
licensed health care professional.

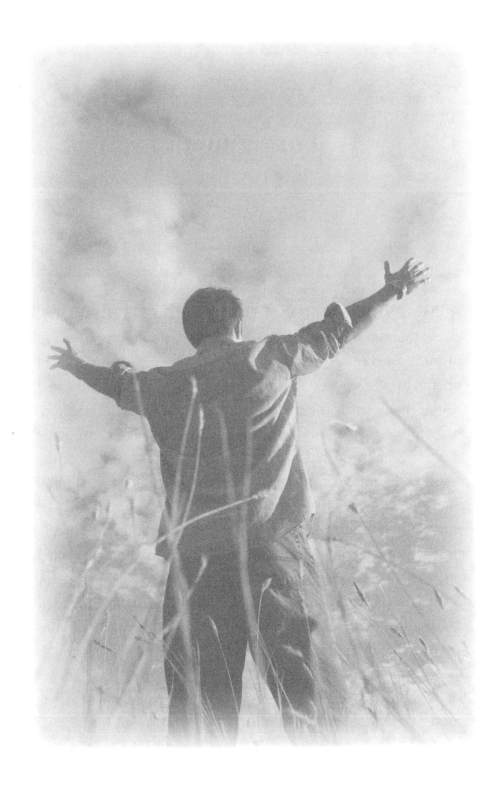

Acknowledgements

THIS BOOK IS DEDICATED TO KAREN, my high school sweetheart and wife of thirty-one years. When God made you He had me in mind, because you make all my dreams come true. Thanks for doing life with me!

This book would not have been possible without my fabulous team at Madeira Chiropractic Wellness Center and Madeira Success Strategies: Missy Markey, Nancy Markey, Joyce Kapp, Linda Plasterer, Amy Haldeman, Dr. Kelli Ross and Dr. J.D. Haynes.

A special thank you to Sarah DelliGatti, whose outstanding talent and creative wisdom made *Fit for the King* so much more than it might have been.

Contents

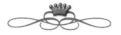

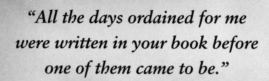

*"All the days ordained for me
were written in your book before
one of them came to be."*

PSALM 139:16

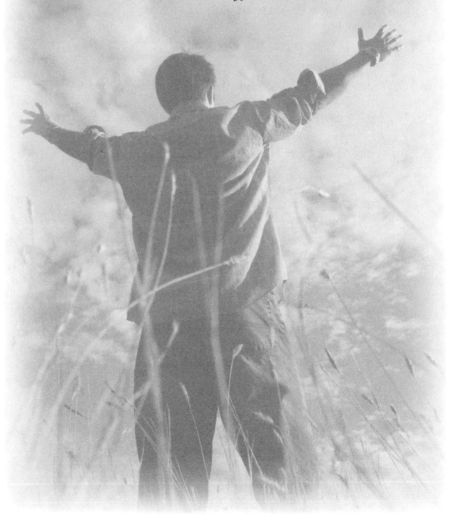

Introduction

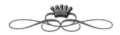

PSALM 139:16 SAYS, "All the days ordained for me were written in your book before one of them came to be." I believe that God ordains a certain number of days for each of us to live here on this earth. I am fully convinced that most people do not live out all of their God-ordained days and that most Christians are not experiencing the quality of life that God desires for them.

My goal for you is that you would live long and strong for Jesus for the rest of your life. I want you to walk in absolute health and well-being your whole life and to die *healthy* at a ripe, old age. Psalm 92:14 says that the righteous, "....will still bear fruit in old age, they will stay fresh and green...." And for what end? So that you are able to accomplish every assignment — both large and small — that the Lord has for you to do. I do not want you to miss one day, one hour, or one divine appointment because you are in pain, sick or suffering from infirmity or disease.

God's word is clear concerning His heart toward us: It is His desire to bless and prosper us in every area of our lives. In Jeremiah 29:11 God states, "For I know the plans I have for you.... plans to prosper you and not to harm you, plans to give you hope and a future."

The purpose of this book is to teach you how to walk in divine health every day of your life. You will be reminded once again what a magnificent creation our bodies are, equipped from birth with the God-given ability to heal themselves. You will discover the true reason that divine health is so vitally important to your calling. You will walk away from each chapter more motivated than ever to take better care of yourself. You will be empowered with the knowledge and wisdom to make divine health a reality instead of a wish in your life. I am privileged to share with you the secrets of nearly three decades of dedication and experience providing natural health care from a Christian perspective to 20,000 different patients.

The end times are closer than ever before and God has much work to be accomplished before Jesus returns. Spectacular health is vital to God's people now more than ever. Every day that your life is cut short by pain, sickness and disease is a day that someone will not hear the gospel or receive the ministry that only you can offer them.

Becoming *Fit for the King* is a choice. It is a decision to place a high priority on your health so that you can be at the ready whenever God needs you to move into action on His behalf.

You have been wonderfully created, lovingly chosen and divinely commissioned to serve in God's kingdom. Come with me on an exciting journey toward divine health and healing and be found *Fit for the King!*

DR. JOHN MADEIRA

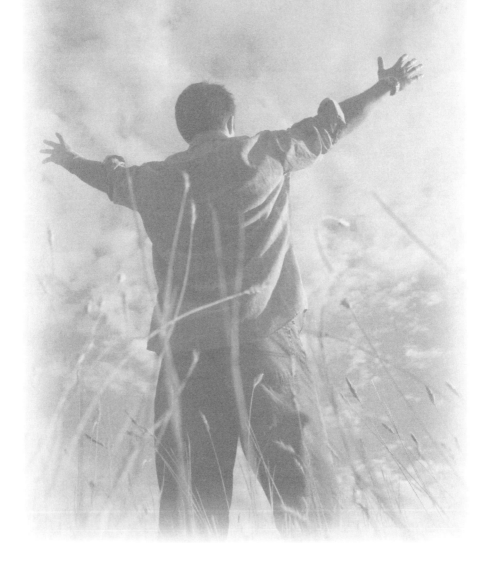

I stand in awe of my body.

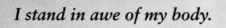

Henry David Thoreau

Chapter One

The Crown *of* His Creation

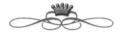

YOU ARE A MASTERPIECE. Your body is more complex than the most technologically advanced piece of machinery ever invented by mankind. Engineers and laborers spend thousands of hours using the most up-to-date, space-age materials to design even the simplest of machines, but God put His first and only prototype in place in moments using the simplest of building materials: dust.

Artists create and recreate, but the most stunning works of art produced are still just a reflection of the most beautiful creation in all of history: the human form.

King David must have been pondering the amazing design of his body when he penned the words of Psalm 139:13-14. "You made all the delicate inner parts of my body and you knit me together in my mother's womb. Thank you for making me so wonderfully complex. Your workmanship is marvelous.

How well I know it." These words were only an echo of God's sentiment, spoken immediately after creating the first man and woman. The work of that day was proclaimed "*very* good."

> **You *are the crown of God's whole creation.***

You are the crown of God's whole creation. No beast of the field, no fish in the sea, not even the mountains towering above the ocean's waves can compare to the creation that you are! God himself has declared it so.

Consider some of the wonderful workings of your body:

Your eye can distinguish 500 different shades of grey. Not just 500 different colors, but 500 different shades of one color! On average, you blink 25 times a minute, without ever thinking about it. More than 8 million times in a year.

God lined your nose with thousands of tiny hairs and a mucous lining to trap the dust you breathe before it gets into your lungs and becomes harmful.

Your ear wax contains a natural insecticide. Did you ever go camping and wonder whether some creepy-crawly might decide your ear would make a cozy home? From the beginning, God put a plan in place to keep those pesky insects from setting up their own camp inside your ear or burrowing to your brain.

Your body contains 600 different muscles, and your tongue is one of the strongest! It's actually a complex set of several muscles that enable you to talk, sing, taste and swallow, and it's covered by ten thousand taste buds.

———⊗⊗⊗———

Your heart beats 100,000 times per day. By the time you're seventy, your heart will have beat 2 ½ billion times.

———⊗⊗⊗———

Your body is filled with a virtual roadmap of arteries and veins, delivering oxygen and nutrients to each cell and picking up waste materials.

———⊗⊗⊗———

Your skeleton consists of 206 different bones, of which the thigh bone is the strongest. Even though they are hollow, your bones are still stronger than concrete.

———⊗⊗⊗———

Your skin is continually being rejuvenated. Every 27 days you shed your outer skin. That is almost 1000 new skins in a lifetime! One square inch of skin has 4 yards of nerve fibers, thirteen-hundred nerve cells, 100 sweat glands, three-million different cells and 3 yards of blood vessels. All are packed into one square inch of skin! Your skin is also the largest organ in your body. It is your first line of defense against germs and disease.

Your heart beats 100,000 times per day.

———⊗⊗⊗———

19

Your body is controlled by its very own personal computer, your brain. Your brain contains one-hundred-billion nerve cells which control and regulate every human function. That three-pound PC generates more electrical impulses in a single day than all of the world's telephones combined. Those nerve impulses travel down the spine and over your nerve system at 270 miles per hour.

Your body contains more than 12 miles of nerves. Every single cell in your body is attached directly or indirectly to your brain via those nerves and responds to the life-giving impulses that travel down those super-highways.

"Your workmanship is marvelous. How well I know it."[1] Even more thrilling than all the parts and pieces is how your body was designed to actually *function*. Each system and organ work seamlessly together, allowing you to live, move, accomplish and dream.

One of the most glorious functions of your body is its built-in ability to heal itself. You cut your finger, it forms a scab. Underneath that ugly, natural band-aid your skin slowly grows back together. Eventually the scab falls off and only a small scar remains. Months later even the scar is gone.

Healing doesn't just take place on your skin, where you can observe it; your body is designed to stay healthy and strong on the inside, too. A virus may sneak past your first lines of

---

1   Psalm 139:14b

defense, but your white blood cells attack and overpower it before it is able to reproduce and wreak havoc on your life.

God truly is an awesome Creator! Not only are you an incredible and beautiful creation, but God programmed your body with a divine ability to heal, repair and rejuvenate itself. As you care for your body, treating it as the very dwelling place of the Holy Spirit, you will experience the divine health that God planned for you when He first formed you in your mother's womb.

> *God programmed your body with a divine ability to heal.*

Lord, thank you for being such an awesome Creator. Thank you for the amazing wisdom and ingenuity that went into creating my body. Your workmanship is truly marvelous! Help me to care for my body so that it will function according to your plan. Thank you that you have given me all I need to walk in divine health. I praise you because I am fearfully and wonderfully made. Amen.

The Crown *of* His Creation
– In Review

- ♛ YOUR BODY IS A MAGNIFICENT CREATION.

- ♛ GOD MADE YOUR BODY WITH A BUILT-IN ABILITY TO HEAL ITSELF.

- ♛ THIS INNATE HEALING MAKES IT POSSIBLE FOR CHRISTIANS TO WALK IN DIVINE HEALTH.

Think of a time when you were sick or injured and reflect on how your body was able to heal itself._____

_____

_____

Imagine what kind of distress people would be in if God had not designed their bodies with an inborn ability to heal. ____

_____

_____

Think back to a time when your body was especially sick or hurting. What circumstances were you dealing with at the time? How were you caring for your body? _____

_____

_____

Now think of a time when your body was especially strong and healthy. Were you making different choices?_____

_____

_____

Can you think of any diet and lifestyle choices that you know would strengthen your body's ability to heal?_____

_____

_____

Notes: _____

_____

_____

_____

_____

_____

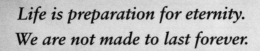

Life is preparation for eternity.
We are not made to last forever.

———

PASTOR RICK WARREN

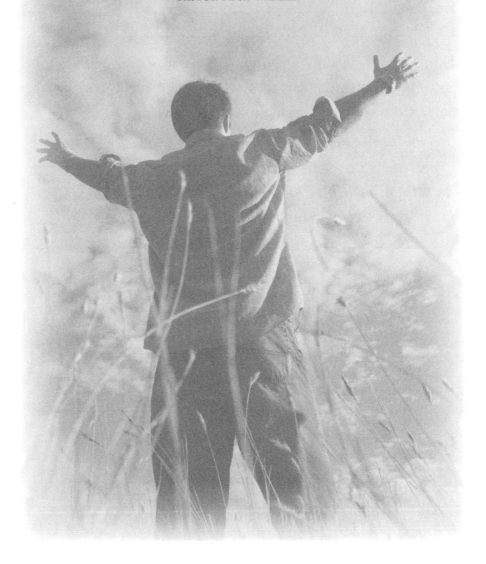

Chapter Two

All the Days Ordained for You

Y OU MAY HAVE HEARD THE SAYING, "God loves
you and has a good plan for your life." That God loves
us is easily understood and generally accepted by most people,
religious or not. But a good plan for our lives? Scripture affirms
this truth over and over with a resounding, "Yes!" Stop for a
moment and consider what God's word says about His plan for
your life:

- ♛ HE KNEW YOU, CALLED YOU AND SET YOU APART BEFORE
  YOU WERE IN YOUR MOTHER'S WOMB. (JEREMIAH 1:5)

- ♛ HIS PLANS FOR YOU ARE GOOD. (JEREMIAH 29:11)

- ♛ HE CHOSE A SPECIFIC TIME AND PLACE FOR YOU TO BE
  BORN AND IMPACT THE WORLD FOR HIS GLORY.
  (ACTS 17:26)

- ♛ EVERY DAY OF YOUR LIFE HAS BEEN ORDAINED (TO
  ESTABLISH OR ORDER BY APPOINTMENT) AND WRITTEN IN

A BOOK; IN FACT, THIS DAUNTING TASK WAS COMPLETED BEFORE YOU WERE EVEN BORN! (PSALM 139:16)

☙ GOD HAS ALREADY PLANNED THE GOOD THINGS YOU CAN ACCOMPLISH WITH YOUR SKILLS, TALENTS AND GIFTS. (EPHESIANS 2:10)

What wonderful reassurance! You and I are not floating through life with no purpose or aim. The God who so marvelously created us also planned the number of our days. His plan is for *our* good and for *His* glory.

> *His plan is for our good and for His glory.*
> ☙

If you consistently make choices to care for and maintain a healthy body, mind and spirit, you will be fully available to live out all the days ordained for you and accomplish all He has planned for you to do. Unfortunately, most people *don't* live out all of those preordained days. In fact, I'm convinced that at least eighty percent of *Christians* die early, before they have had a chance to enjoy all of the days God has planned for them.

Seventy-eight percent of Americans suffer and die from preventable illnesses, too often the result of result of destructive choices. Each destructive choice accumulates and the consequences over time cause illness, disease and death. Too many of our ordained days are filled with sickness and pain, which easily shifts our focus from God's plan to simply surviving.

> *Seventy-eight percent of Americans suffer and die from preventable illnesses.*
> ☙

Even if disease does not claim our life early, we stumble through our days without the fullness of joy and abundant life that God intended. Others do succumb to disease and die early, never experiencing the richness and length of days that God had planned for them. How many grandparents were supposed to be giant spiritual leaders in the lives of their grandchildren if cancer or another illness had not claimed them years before those precious babies were even born? How many non-Christians might have been brought to the Lord by a mature Christian who did not walk out the fullness of their days due to obesity-related diabetes? Brothers and sisters, there is a better way! When we make a conscious choice to care for our bodies we partner with God, giving our bodies all they need to heal and stay strong and healthy, empowering them to fulfill every purpose and plan of God's until the last breath we take.

There are hundreds of great reasons to maintain a healthy body, including freedom from pain, ease of movement, increased energy and elevated mood to name just a few. But if you are a Christian, those pale in comparison to the real benefits of good health. Your body will be able to live each day walking in God's will, doing His work, bringing Him glory, resulting in a life filled with the fruit of His Spirit. Lower blood pressure, lower cholesterol, balanced blood sugar and freedom from disease are all wonderful benefits to be thankful for, but the true treasure is a life lived "long and strong for Jesus."

> *True treasure is a life lived "long and strong for Jesus."*

This motivation for good health is the greatest one of all because it makes daily decisions incredibly simple. "God has plans for me today. I will make healthy choices and partner with Him for my good and His glory."

Too often, our goals of lowering cholesterol or losing 20 pounds have little impact on the choices we are making as we pull into the drive-thru at a fast food place. But if we consider that a double cheeseburger may impact our ability to serve God *today* and that a double cheeseburger *habit* will certainly impact us negatively over a course of years, the decision to stay healthy is much simpler. Will you steward yourself and maintain a healthy body that will survive to fulfill his plans for your life up until that last, glorious day when He calls you home?

There are two primary reasons that people die before those days have been completed. The first is a lack of knowledge. You simply might not know *how* to take good care of your body. Perhaps you grew up in a family where maintaining good health was never a priority. Maybe you were simply never taught to consider the long-term consequences of daily decisions.

The second reason people die early is a lack of discipline. You might already know *how* to take care of your body; you just lack the self-discipline to actually *do* it. In our country, I believe most people fall into this latter category. *Someone* is buying all those health magazines at the grocery checkout, but a quick glance at the folks in line will confirm that not too many of us are actually putting the knowledge into practice!

The good news is there is help! If you are lacking knowledge, this book will lead you in the right direction. The following chapters are filled with information and practical steps to help you "live long and strong for Jesus." If you lack discipline, I have just given you the best motivation in the world for putting what you know into practice: to live out every day God has ordained for you. God does love you, and He does have a good plan for your life. You don't want to miss a day of it!

You are not alone in your journey to better health. The God who created you so masterfully, who has plans for each day of your life, also gives power by his Holy Spirit to help you make wise choices and to be disciplined. God cares about your health and He wants to guide and direct you! The Bible says that you can ask Him for wisdom, and He won't scoff at your request.[2] Ask Him today!

God, thank you that your plans for me are good. Thank you that you created my body to live long and strong to fulfill your plans and purposes in my life. I don't want to miss a single day! I pray a covering of health and healing over myself and my loved ones, and I rebuke every attack of the enemy against my body that would keep me from living out every day you have ordained for me. Thank you that I'm not alone, that you are walking with me, giving me the strength, willpower and resolve to make good choices. I want to glorify you every day of my life. Amen.

---

2   If any of you lacks wisdom, he should ask God, who gives generously to all without finding fault, and it will be given to him. James 1:5

All the Days Ordained for You
– In Review

- ♛ NOTHING ABOUT YOU IS ACCIDENTAL. GOD CREATED YOU WITH A SPECIFIC PLAN FOR YOUR LIFE THAT WAS ALREADY MAPPED OUT AND RECORDED BEFORE YOUR BIRTH.

- ♛ IF YOU TAKE CARE OF YOUR BODY YOU WILL LIVE OUT EVERY PRE-ORDAINED DAY THAT GOD PLANNED FOR YOU.

- ♛ IF YOU DO NOT TAKE CARE OF YOUR BODY, YOU RISK DYING BEFORE ALL OF YOUR ORDAINED DAYS HAVE BEEN COMPLETED.

- ♛ EVEN IF YOU DO NOT DIE EARLY, SICKNESS AND DISEASE CAN KEEP YOU FROM LIVING THE WONDERFUL LIFE THAT GOD PLANNED FOR YOU.

- ♛ CHRISTIANS DIE BEFORE THEIR APPOINTED TIME EITHER BECAUSE THEY LACK KNOWLEDGE ABOUT HOW TO PROPERLY CARE FOR THEIR BODIES OR BECAUSE THEY LACK THE DISCIPLINE NEEDED TO CARE FOR THEIR BODIES.

- ♛ THE BEST MOTIVATION FOR TAKING GOOD CARE OF YOUR BODY IS SO THAT YOU WILL BE ABLE TO LIVE EVERY DAY GOD PLANNED FOR YOU TO THE FULLEST.

Have you known a Christian who seemed to die too early, before they had walked out what you believed to be their God-ordained calling? _____

_____

_____

What has motivated you to pursue good health in the past? The scale? Your high blood pressure or high cholesterol? Were those things enough to keep you on track? _____

_____

_____

Have you ever considered that the most important reason for pursuing good health is to enable you to live all of the days God ordained for you? _____

_____

_____

If you have had family members die of sickness and disease, how old were they? If you die at about the same age as your parents or grandparents did, will you be satisfied that you lived a long, healthy life? _____

_____

_____

Notes: _____

_____

_____

_____

_____

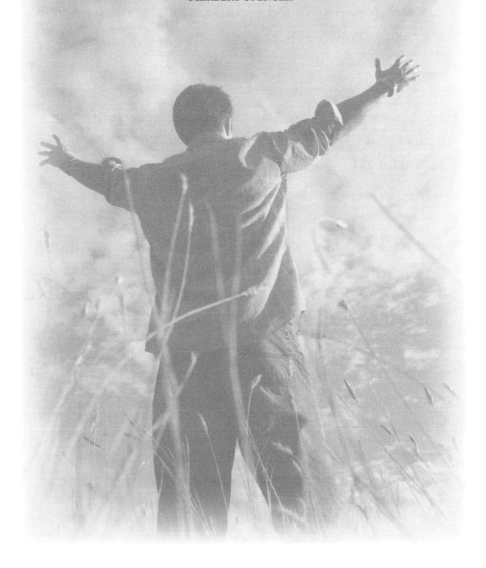

The preservation of health is a duty.

⊸∞∞⊷

HERBERT SPENCER

Chapter Three

God Wants You to Walk in Divine Health

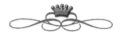

YOU ARE THE CROWN OF GOD'S CREATION, and God has a wonderful plan for each and every day of your life. With those wonderful foundations firmly in place, it is time to believe another daring truth: God wants you to walk in *divine* health.

"Divine" simply means that something is supremely good because it proceeds directly from God. Most people have never stopped to consider that a healthy, fully functioning body is the supremely good plan of God for their life! When you boil it all down, your health is your single greatest asset because without it, nothing else matters.

Your health is your single greatest asset.

Let's consider what divine health might look like in the life of a believer.

- ♛ SICKNESS IS RARE
- ♛ REFRESHING, DEEP SLEEP IS THE NORM
- ♛ FREEDOM FROM PAIN
- ♛ NO USE OF PRESCRIPTION OR OVER-THE-COUNTER MEDICATIONS
- ♛ HIGH ENERGY LEVELS
- ♛ A HEALTHY SEX DRIVE
- ♛ GREAT POSTURE
- ♛ NEVER HOSPITALIZED
- ♛ GREAT APPETITE WITHOUT FOOD CRAVINGS
- ♛ AN EMPTY MEDICINE CABINET
- ♛ A CONSISTENT, JOYFUL ATTITUDE
- ♛ YOUTHFUL, VIBRANT APPEARANCE
- ♛ NORMAL CHOLESTEROL
- ♛ NORMAL BLOOD PRESSURE
- ♛ NO ARTHRITIC CONDITIONS
- ♛ REGULAR BOWEL MOVEMENTS
- ♛ TRIM AND FIT
- ♛ BALANCED HORMONES
- ♛ SURGERY-FREE
- ♛ HEALTHY SKIN

Of course, these are only some of the characteristics of divine health. Scripture says that signs and wonders should follow Christians. If every Christian walked around in divine health these characteristics would be powerful "signs" of God's goodness and truth to our sick and hurting world. Imagine what a witness it would be to the world if Christians were the healthiest people on the planet!

I can personally attest to the wonderful blessing of divine health. I have been living the principles contained in this book for the past 36 years. In all of that time, I have only been sick enough to need prescription medication *once,* which I took for the full ten days as prescribed. I have never undergone surgery or had any reason to be admitted to a hospital.

Unfortunately, too many people (Christians included) cannot relate to that wonderful list. In fact, I am often amazed when attending church services at the number of hands that go up when the pastor asks who is in need of prayer for physical healing. There is certainly nothing wrong with admitting that you need a brother or sister to pray for you, but too often it seems that 75 percent of the congregation is in need of healing from pain or disease. It grieves my heart because I know that there is a better way. Too often, Christians identify more with these characteristics of "dis-ease:"

- ☙ CHRONIC FATIGUE OR LOW ENERGY
- ☙ WAKING UP TIRED IS THE NORM
- ☙ RECURRING HEADACHES
- ☙ OVERWEIGHT OR OBESE
- ☙ CHRONIC PAIN OR TENSION IN THE NECK AND/OR BACK
- ☙ ALLERGIES AND/OR SINUS PROBLEMS

- ♛ CHRONIC BREATHING PROBLEMS, ASTHMA, COPD

- ♛ CHRONIC CONSTIPATION, HEMORRHOIDS

- ♛ IRRITABLE BOWEL SYNDROME, COLITIS OR CHRONIC DIGESTIVE PROBLEMS

- ♛ REGULAR USE OF PRESCRIPTION MEDICATIONS

- ♛ IRRITABILITY AND MOOD SWINGS

- ♛ A PROTRUDING BELLY

- ♛ CHRONIC BAD BREATH AND/OR BODY ODOR

- ♛ FOUL-SMELLING STOOLS, EXCESSIVE GAS

- ♛ SUGAR CRAVINGS

- ♛ FREQUENT ILLNESS

- ♛ CHRONIC SKIN RASHES OR SKIN IRRITATIONS

- ♛ POOR POSTURE

- ♛ HIGH BLOOD SUGAR

- ♛ FREQUENT DOCTOR VISITS

- ♛ HIGH CHOLESTEROL

- ♛ LOW OR ABSENT SEX DRIVE, ERECTILE DYSFUNCTION

- ♛ HISTORY OF MULTIPLE HOSPITAL STAYS AND/OR MULTIPLE SURGERIES

- ♛ REGULAR USE OF PAIN RELIEVERS OR OTHER OVER-THE-COUNTER MEDICINE

These are just some of the signs and symptoms that you are not walking in the level of divine health that God has made available. Do any of them resonate with you? Jesus said, "I have come that they may have life, and that they may have it more abundantly."[3] Does this sound like the abundant life He promised His people?

> "I have come that they may have life, and that they may have it more abundantly."
>
> ♛

Sometimes the truth is upsetting, but the unpleasant realization that we are not walking in a level of divine health can also be a strong catalyst for change. Once we make an honest assessment of our present level of health, the truth really *can* set us free to make changes that will result in divine health.

If you are unsure about your level of health after reading both lists, consider talking with a friend, a family member, or a trusted health care provider. Ask God to reveal your true level of health through any of these sources so that you can start taking steps to even greater divine health. And don't be discouraged! Satan is our accuser and he would love for you to put this book away right now in discouragement and shame. Remind him that the Holy Spirit living within you has made you "more than a conqueror"[4] over ill health and disease and that you are not under condemnation but under grace and loving-kindness!

If you are walking in high levels of divine health, praise the Lord! And if you see areas for improvement, praise the Lord as well. By taking an honest assessment of your health, you have

---

3   John 10:10, NKJ

4   "....in all these things we are more than conquerors through him who loved us." Romans 8:37

taken the first crucial step in living long and strong for Jesus. It is an exciting adventure that we will explore more fully in the coming chapters.

> D*ear Father, thank you that through you my health can improve. Help me to walk in a greater level of divine health. Thank you for helping me to take an honest look at how my body is functioning and where changes are needed to live long and strong for you. Thank you that I am not alone on this journey, but that you are walking next to me every step of the way. Reveal to me those places where I need to make changes, help me to be more disciplined and may my increasing health only bring more and more glory to your name each day. Amen.*

God Wants You to Walk in Divine Health – In Review

- ☫ DIVINE HEALTH PROCEEDS DIRECTLY FROM GOD AS WE CARE FOR OUR BODIES AS HE INTENDED.

- ☫ CHRISTIANS WALKING IN DIVINE HEALTH ARE A "SIGN AND WONDER" OF GOD'S POWER TO UNBELIEVERS.

- ☫ THE LIFE LIVED IN DIVINE HEALTH IS VIBRANT, JOYFUL AND PAIN-FREE.

- ☫ UNFORTUNATELY, MOST CHRISTIANS ARE NOT WALKING IN DIVINE HEALTH.

- ☫ THE LIFE THAT LACKS DIVINE HEALTH WILL ULTIMATELY BE OVERTAKEN WITH SICKNESS, DISEASE AND SUFFERING.

- ☫ IT IS IMPORTANT TO HAVE AN HONEST ASSESSMENT OF YOUR HEALTH SO THAT CHANGES CAN BE MADE.

- ☫ GOD WANTS EVERY SINGLE ONE OF HIS PEOPLE TO WALK IN DIVINE HEALTH.

How would you rate your level of health on a scale of one to ten (ten being the best)? _____

_____

_____

Would you call your present level of health "divine health?"_

_____

_____

Are you aware of important areas of your life that are being neglected because you are suffering from poor health? _____

_____

_____

What dreams and goals would you strive for if divine health made you more able to pursue them?_____

_____

_____

Notes: _____

_____

_____

_____

_____

_____

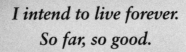

I intend to live forever.
So far, so good.

STEVEN WRIGHT

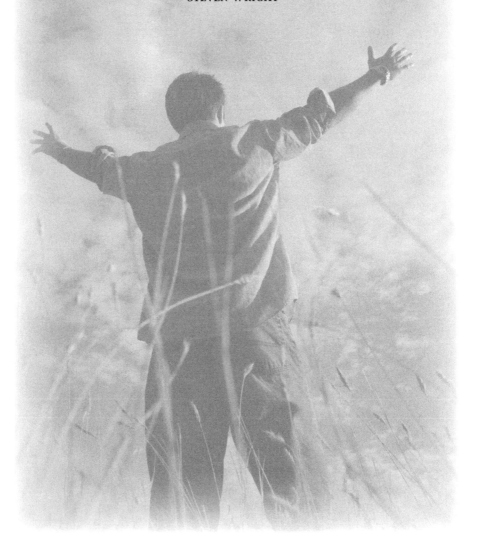

Chapter Four

An Honest Self-Assessment

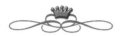

A N HONEST SELF-ASSESSMENT will help you determine your present level of health and what changes can be made to achieve a greater level of divine health.

Check all that apply to you:

LIST A

❑ I RARELY GET SICK.

❑ MOST NIGHTS I GET REFRESHING, DEEP SLEEP.

❑ I RARELY EXPERIENCE PAIN IN MY BODY.

❑ I DON'T TAKE MEDICATION.

❑ MY ENERGY LEVELS ARE HIGH.

❑ I HAVE A HEALTHY SEX DRIVE.

❑ I HAVE GOOD POSTURE.

❑ I HAVE HAD NO HOSPITAL STAYS.

❑ I HAVE A GREAT APPETITE AND DO NOT EXPERIENCE FOOD CRAVINGS.

❑ MY MEDICINE CABINET IS EMPTY.

❑ I HAVE A CONSISTENT, JOYFUL ATTITUDE.

❑ I LOOK YOUNG FOR MY AGE.

❑ MY CHOLESTEROL LEVELS ARE NORMAL.

❑ I HAVE NORMAL BLOOD PRESSURE LEVELS.

❑ I DON'T SUFFER FROM ANY ARTHRITIC CONDITIONS.

❑ I HAVE REGULAR BOWEL MOVEMENTS.

❑ I EXERCISE FREQUENTLY.

❑ MY HORMONES ARE BALANCED.

❑ I DON'T KNOW OF ANY NEED FOR SURGERY.

❑ MY SKIN IS HEALTHY AND YOUTHFUL FOR MY AGE.

LIST B

❑ I'M OFTEN FATIGUED AND HAVE LITTLE ENERGY.

❑ I'M STILL TIRED WHEN I WAKE UP IN THE MORNING.

❑ I HAVE RECURRING HEADACHES.

❑ I AM OVERWEIGHT OR OBESE.

❑ I SUFFER FROM CHRONIC PAIN OR TENSION.

❑ I HAVE CHRONIC ALLERGIES AND/OR SINUS PROBLEMS.

❑ I HAVE CHRONIC BREATHING PROBLEMS, ASTHMA OR COPD.

❑ I'M CHRONICALLY CONSTIPATED AND/OR HAVE HEMORRHOIDS.

❑ I HAVE IRRITABLE BOWEL SYNDROME, COLITIS OR CHRONIC DIGESTIVE CHALLENGES.

❑ I REGULARLY USE PRESCRIPTION OR OVER-THE-COUNTER MEDICATIONS.

❑ I'M OFTEN IRRITABLE AND MOODY.

❑ I HAVE A PROTRUDING BELLY.

❑ I HAVE CHRONIC BAD BREATH AND/OR BODY ODOR.

❑ MY STOOLS HAVE A FOUL SMELL AND/OR I HAVE EXCESSIVE GAS.

❑ I OFTEN CRAVE SUGAR AND SWEETS.

❑ I'M FREQUENTLY SICK.

❑ I HAVE CHRONIC SKIN RASHES OR SKIN IRRITATIONS.

❑ I HAVE POOR POSTURE.

❑ I HAVE HIGH BLOOD SUGAR.

❑ I MAKE FREQUENT TRIPS TO THE DOCTOR FOR SICKNESS OR PAIN.

❑ I HAVE HIGH CHOLESTEROL.

❑ I HAVE A LOW OR ABSENT SEX DRIVE.

❑ I CAN'T ACHIEVE AND/OR MAINTAIN AN ERECTION

❑ I'VE HAD MULTIPLE HOSPITAL STAYS AND/OR MULTIPLE SURGERIES.

❑ I USE PAIN RELIEVERS OR OTHER OVER-THE-COUNTER MEDICINES REGULARLY.

List A is full of the signs of those who walk in divine health. If you find yourself checking more of the symptoms in List B, I have good news. This book will teach you many practical ways to gain victory over your health issues and begin walking in the levels of health God desires for you.

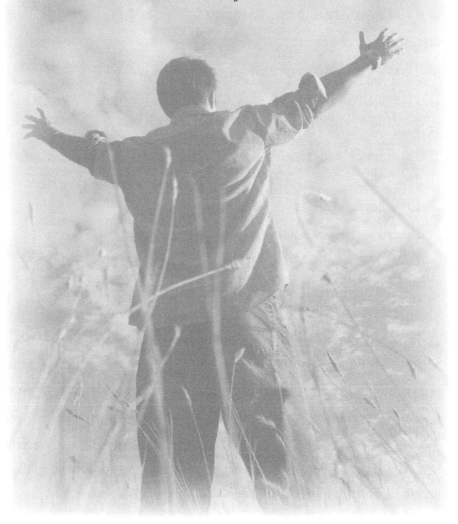

A man seldom thinks with more earnestness of anything than he does of his dinner.

DR. SAMUEL JOHNSON

Chapter Five

Foods that Empower, Foods that Devour

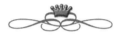

I AM SURE YOU HAVE HEARD the old adage, "You are what you eat." What you might not realize is that it is absolutely true!

Your body is made up of trillions of cells. These cells are clumped together to form tissues and organs that perform specific functions.

Cells have a lifespan of about 90-120 days before dying. Because your body is so wonderfully designed, it recycles any reusable parts from old cells and discards what remains. Brand new cells are continually and efficiently produced to replace the ones that die — and all this without one conscious thought on your part! The primary building material for this huge endeavor? It is the food that you eat every day.

Imagine for a moment that you decide to build a new house. You hire a builder, who starts the project by constructing a foundation. Whether it's a concrete slab or cinderblock walls, he knows that the full weight of your new home will rest upon this hidden foundation. Any weakness or shifting will jeopardize the stability of the entire structure.

In the same way, your diet is the foundation of your health, affecting each tiny cell that makes up every tissue and organ. What you put into your mouth is the raw building material that will be used to construct either strong, efficient tissues or weak, sickly ones. And because your cells only last 3 to 6 months before dying and being replaced, you have an entirely new body once or twice a year! That's encouraging news, because just a few months of providing good nutritional building materials will make a marked difference in your level of health.

Constructive Versus Destructive Food

Foods are either constructive or destructive in their effects on your health and well-being. If you consistently eat constructive foods that provide what your body needs to build strong, vibrant cells, your body will be empowered to "live long and strong for Jesus."[5] When you consume destructive foods on a regular basis, cells are built with second-rate building materials and tissues and organs become foundationally weak. We set ourselves up for disease over the long term and are literally opening the door for the devil to steal our health.

---

[5]   "Don't you realize that your body is the temple of the Holy Spirit, who lives in you and was given to you by God? You do not belong to yourself." 1 Corinthians 6:19

Prior to World War II, the quality of our food supply was far superior to what is available now. Diets were comprised of "whole" foods that were grown on local farms without harsh chemicals and pesticides. Mothers prepared most of the meals in the family kitchen from scratch.

Many folks nostalgically think back to those "good old days" of family dinners and home cooking. Today we are much more likely to open a box of processed food that was prepared with high tech machinery for mass consumption. Microwaveable frozen meals and canned food seem to meet the needs of our busy schedules. Fruits and vegetables are picked before they are ripe so they can be shipped long distances.[6]

Eating has never been so easy – or so dangerous to our health.

Grains, fruits and vegetables are genetically modified, grown with harsh chemicals and radiated before they reach the grocery shelf. Meat, fish and dairy products such as eggs and milk are produced on large farms where animals are routinely fed antibiotics and are injected with hormones for faster growth and higher production.

If we are especially busy or the cupboards are bare, there is always a fast food drive-thru willing to "supersize" the fries and diet soda that come with our value meal. (Some value!) Eating has never been so easy – or so dangerous to our health.

---

6   Much of our fruit and vegetable supplies are grown in Central and South American countries.

The processing, refining and mechanization of our food supply has become a kind of "nutritional suicide."

So how do we eat well in the midst of our high paced lifestyles? I doubt that you have time to grow and manage your own garden or raise hormone-free beef cattle in your backyard. But there *are* ways to eat well and raise a healthy family in the 21st century, and it all starts with becoming informed and making wise choices.

Live Foods versus Dead Foods

Our first rule is to eat live foods instead of dead foods. Live foods were recently alive, either as an animal or growing on a tree, bush or in the ground. Examples include eggs, fresh meats, fruits and vegetables.

Divine health requires a firm foundation of healthy, live foods.

Dead foods are processed foods and typically come in a box, can or mechanically-sealed wrapper. Examples include white flour, commercial cereals, candies, cake mixes, prepared meals and canned fruits and vegetables. These dead foods usually come with a long ingredient list that includes preservatives, additives, food colorings and words that most of us cannot even pronounce. This leads us to a good second rule to follow when making food choices: If you can't pronounce it, you probably shouldn't eat it!

Our third guideline is that typically the shorter the ingredients list, the healthier a food is for you. Becoming a label reader will help you make healthier food choices.

Simply stated, divine health requires a firm foundation of healthy, live foods. You wouldn't use faulty building materials and then be angry when a violent storm blew your new house down. In the same way, you can't feed your body a steady diet of destructive foods and expect it to battle illness and disease when they come knocking at your door.

If you are starting to connect the dots between your diet and health problems, don't be discouraged. The following chapters will further explain how choosing healthy, constructive foods will bring you to a new level of divine health that you have probably only dreamed of. Join me on this exciting journey as we take steps to "live long and strong for Jesus."

Thank you, Lord, that you have provided all of the good, constructive food that I need to build a foundation of health and healing in my body. I am grateful that you are opening my eyes to better choices and a better way of living. Please give me continued insight and the strength to make changes that will propel me to even greater levels of divine health. May my body live long and strong for you. Amen.

Foods the Empower, Foods that Devour – In Review

- ✠ YOUR BODY IS CONSTANTLY REBUILDING ITSELF CELL BY CELL.

- ✠ THE RAW MATERIAL YOUR BODY USES TO REBUILD ITSELF COMES DIRECTLY FROM THE FOOD THAT YOU EAT.

- ✠ FOODS ARE EITHER CONSTRUCTIVE OR DESTRUCTIVE TO YOUR BODY.

- ✠ CONSUMING DESTRUCTIVE, UNHEALTHY FOOD WILL RESULT IN AN UNHEALTHY BODY THAT CANNOT HEAL ITSELF AS GOD INTENDED.

- ✠ CONSUMING CONSTRUCTIVE, HEALTHY FOOD WILL RESULT IN A HEALTHY BODY THAT IS ABLE TO HEAL ITSELF AS GOD INTENDED.

- ✠ "LIVE FOODS" ARE MADE BY GOD. THEY WERE ONCE ALIVE, EITHER AS AN ANIMAL, IN THE GROUND OR ON A TREE OR BUSH. THESE FOODS ARE GENERALLY CONSTRUCTIVE FOODS.

- ✠ "DEAD FOODS" ARE MAN-MADE, PROCESSED FOODS THAT ARE PACKAGED IN BOXES AND CANS. THESE FOODS ARE GENERALLY DESTRUCTIVE FOODS.

- ✠ THREE USEFUL RULES TO FOLLOW ARE:
    1. EAT LIVE FOODS INSTEAD OF DEAD FOODS.
    2. IF AN INGREDIENT LIST IS FULL OF WORDS YOU CANNOT PRONOUNCE, DO NOT EAT IT.
    3. GENERALLY SPEAKING THE SHORTER AN INGREDIENT LIST IS, THE BETTER THE FOOD IS FOR YOUR BODY.

- ✠ DIVINE HEALTH REQUIRES A FIRM FOUNDATION OF HEALTHY, LIVE FOODS

If you are at home, take a quick peak inside your pantry and refrigerator. Would you say that the foods they contain are mostly constructive or destructive?_____

_____

_____

Think of the restaurants you frequently visit. Do they generally offer constructive or destructive foods? _____

_____

_____

Go grab your favorite snack and read through the ingredients list out loud. Do you need to reconsider a healthier alternative? _____

_____

_____

Notes: _____

_____

_____

_____

_____

_____

_____

_____

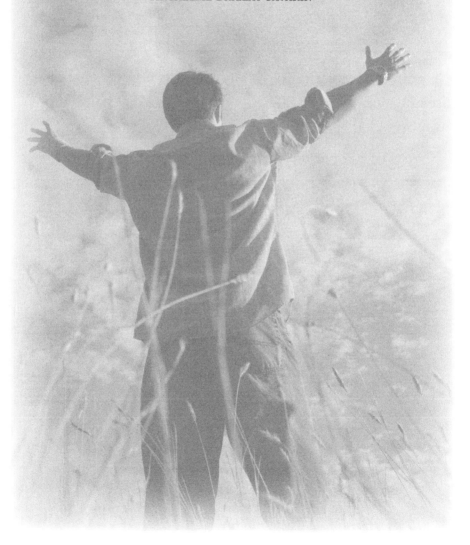

Tell me what you eat,
and I will tell you what you are.

———✦———

ANTHELME BRILLAT-SAVARIN

Chapter Six

What's In a Label?

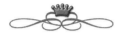

IT IS IMPORTANT TO MAKE WISE CHOICES when choosing what foods to purchase for you and your family. Understanding nutrition labels will help you know exactly what is in a particular food so that you can either eat it joyfully or leave it on the grocer's shelf.

The U.S. Food and Drug Administration (USFDA) has adopted a nutrition label that is used consistently by food manufacturers.

The label consists of five basic areas:

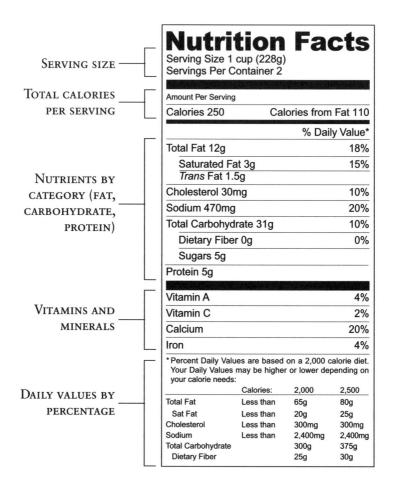

SERVING SIZE

TOTAL CALORIES
PER SERVING

NUTRIENTS BY
CATEGORY (FAT,
CARBOHYDRATE,
PROTEIN)

VITAMINS AND
MINERALS

DAILY VALUES BY
PERCENTAGE

Nutrition Facts

Serving Size 1 cup (228g)
Servings Per Container 2

Amount Per Serving

Calories 250   Calories from Fat 110

% Daily Value*

Total Fat 12g	18%
Saturated Fat 3g	15%
Trans Fat 1.5g	
Cholesterol 30mg	10%
Sodium 470mg	20%
Total Carbohydrate 31g	10%
Dietary Fiber 0g	0%
Sugars 5g	
Protein 5g	

Vitamin A	4%
Vitamin C	2%
Calcium	20%
Iron	4%

* Percent Daily Values are based on a 2,000 calorie diet.
Your Daily Values may be higher or lower depending on
your calorie needs:

	Calories:	2,000	2,500
Total Fat	Less than	65g	80g
Sat Fat	Less than	20g	25g
Cholesterol	Less than	300mg	300mg
Sodium	Less than	2,400mg	2,400mg
Total Carbohydrate		300g	375g
Dietary Fiber		25g	30g

When reviewing a nutrition label, start by determining the serving size first. All of the nutrition information on the label is listed per serving. For example, if the serving size is 8 pretzels and the label states that one serving contains 175 calories, it means there are 175 calories in 8 pretzels. Always ask yourself, "How many servings do I intend to consume?" and determine how many calories that will be. The number of servings you eat determines the number of calories and nutrition you are getting. Carefully considering the serving size and total calories will help you control portion sizes. Controlling portion sizes is one of the hallmark decisions of every person who wants to remain "Fit for the King."

Do not consume foods that contain trans fats.

The next area to consider is the total fat in each serving. High fat diets, especially those high in saturated fat, have been linked to higher rates of cancer. Fats are necessary for proper function of our bodies. People who eat leaner (less fat) diets are typically thinner than their counterparts. You should especially limit your intake of saturated (animal) fat. Olive oil is a wonderful, healthy replacement. In addition, do not consume foods that contain trans fats. As we have already discussed, trans fats are chemically modified and have been shown to cause cancer, raise bad cholesterol and lower good cholesterol.

After you consider the fat in a serving, take a look at cholesterol and sodium levels. This is especially important if you have high cholesterol, heart problems, high blood pressure or a history of heart attacks or heart disease.

Only 25 percent of Americans get enough fiber in their diets.

Now look at the fiber content of the food product you are considering. Only 25 percent of Americans get enough fiber in their diets, despite the fact that a high-fiber diet lowers cholesterol, lowers the risk of bowel and colon cancer, helps prevent constipation and helps the body remove toxins and poisons from the intestines.

Also listed in this area of the nutrition label is total sugar and carbohydrate content. The more sugar and carbohydrates in a food the faster it will digest in your body. This is called a food's "glycemic index." These types of foods cause a quick increase in blood sugar and precipitate the quick release of insulin known as "insulin response." Insulin is a hormone secreted by your pancreas which lowers blood sugar when it gets too high. Insulin tells the body's cells to take in sugar from the blood and use it either for energy or to store it for future use. If you do not need energy at the moment (for exercise or physical labor, for example), the calories will be stored as.... fat. This is another reason that it is important to be aware of the number of calories you are consuming and to control the size of your portions.

There are 76 ways white refined sugar can ruin your health.

Keep in mind that the sugars listed include both naturally occurring sugar (from fruit, for example) as well as added sugars such as white, refined sugar or high fructose corn syrup. You will need to refer to the ingredients list to determine what type of sugars the food contains.

According to Nancy Appleton, PhD., author of *Lick the Sugar Habit*, there are 76 ways white refined sugar can ruin your health. In my opinion, as well as many other health experts, sugar and high fructose corn syrup are responsible for most of the obesity and diabetes occurring in the U.S.[7]

The next area of the nutrition label lists the vitamins and minerals the food contains. Obviously, the more nutrient-rich a food is, the better it is for you. You will quickly realize as you pay closer attention to this area of the label why it is important to take nutrition supplements. You will also quickly come to agree that you need more food in your diet grown by Mother Nature versus manufactured by a food processing plant. The nutritional value of man-made food pales in comparison to God-made food every time!

The final part of the Nutrition Facts label to consider is the Daily Values, labeled as %DV or Percentage of Daily Value. These numbers are listed on the far right column of the food label. This percentage helps you determine the percent of the total recommended daily amount for each specific nutrient.

Let me explain. If calcium is listed under the vitamin and mineral area as being 20 percent of the %DV (daily value)[8], then consuming 1 serving of that particular food would give you 20 percent of the recommended daily amount for calcium. If you were to consume five servings of this food in a day you would get 100 percent of the recommended daily amount for calcium.

Most nutrition facts labels include only the information we just covered. When a food's packaging is large enough, you will often see a footnote area across the bottom of the label which

---

7   Two thirds of all U.S. adults are significantly overweight. Approximately 1/3 of all US adults are considered obese.

8   %DVs are based on an average 2000 calorie per day diet.

lists reference information for the Percent Daily Values for total fat, saturated fat, cholesterol, sodium, total carbohydrates and dietary fiber. This information can be a helpful reminder of how many grams of a nutrient you should be eating every day or how much saturated fat per day is considered unhealthy.

Another very important method of evaluating the merits of a food product is the ingredients list. While it is not officially a part of the nutrition facts label, the FDA requires that ingredients be listed. It is important to realize that the ingredients in a product are listed in descending order of quantity. In other words, the ingredient listed first makes up the highest percentage of the product's total ingredients. The ingredient listed last makes up the smallest percentage of total ingredients.

Most pretzels, for example, are made up primarily of wheat flour, salt, yeast and soda. Wheat flour is the primary ingredient and soda is the smallest quantity of ingredient used. The ingredients list does not tell you exactly how much of each ingredient is used but does give you an indication simply by the order in which ingredients are listed.

Some other helpful food facts you should consider:

- ⚜ MANUFACTURERS ARE NOT REQUIRED TO DISCLOSE WHAT KIND OF FLAVORINGS A PRODUCT CONTAINS, JUST THAT IT CONTAINS THEM (IE. NATURAL VERSUS ARTIFICIAL FLAVOR).

- ⚜ THE LONGER AN INGREDIENT LIST IS, THE LESS HEALTHY A FOOD TENDS TO BE (WITH EXCEPTIONS).

- ⚜ "NO TRANS FAT" LISTED ON THE FRONT PACKAGING OF A FOOD DOES NOT NECESSARILY MEAN IT CONTAINS ZERO TRANS FAT. THE FDA ALLOWS FOOD MANUFACTURERS TO

LABEL A FOOD "NO TRANS FAT" IF THERE IS LESS THEN .5
GRAMS OF TRANS FAT PER SERVING.

☙ TRANS FAT IS USUALLY IDENTIFIED IN THE INGREDIENT
LIST AS "PARTIALLY HYDROGENATED" OIL, USUALLY
SOYBEAN OR COTTONSEED OIL. DO NOT PURCHASE OR
CONSUME PRODUCTS CONTAINING TRANS FAT.

☙ SUGAR IS OFTEN DISGUISED IN FOOD INGREDIENT LISTS
AS DEXTROSE, SUCROSE, HIGH FRUCTOSE CORN SYRUP,
MALTOSE, FRUCTOSE AND EVAPORATED CANE JUICE.
(NOTICE THAT MOST OF THE CHEMICAL NAMES FOR SUGAR
END IN "-OSE.")

Take this short quiz to see what you have learned about
nutrition fact labels and ingredient listings:

1. *A food is listed as having a serving size of one ounce. The
   servings per bag is 16 ounces. How many total ounces are in
   the bag?*

2. *If a food label states that a product contains 25% DV (daily
   value) of fiber per serving, how many servings would you
   have to eat in a day to get 100 percent of the recommended
   daily amount?*

3. *If a serving size of two chocolate cookies equals 250
   calories and you eat 4 cookies, how many calories have you
   consumed?*

4. *If you have high blood pressure, heart disease, high
   cholesterol or have had a heart attack, which nutrients
   should you pay particular attention to?*

5. *If you are constipated or have cholesterol problems or you
   want to lower your risk of bowel or colon cancer you should
   be sure to pay special attention to what food ingredient?*

6. *What is a hallmark habit of people who maintain a healthy weight and want to be "Fit for the King"?*

7. *When you eat too many calories at one time your body will produce what hormone and for what purpose?*

8. *When your body stores excess energy from eating too many calories at one time, that food will be stored as what?*

9. *What food ingredient is the most deadly when you consider the diseases that are caused by consistently consuming it in large quantities?*

Answers: (1) 16 oz. (2) 4 servings (3) 500 calories (4) total fat, saturated fat, trans fat, cholesterol, sodium (5) fiber (6) portion size (7) insulin to lower blood sugar levels (8) fat (9) refined sugar and high fructose corn syrup

Nutrition fact labels and ingredient lists are a wonderful tool that will help you make wiser food choices. It has been my experience that food even *tastes* better when you know exactly what you are eating and how good it is for your body! Make wise food choices and start enjoying new levels of energy and health today.

Lord, thank you that food is so readily available to me. Help me to make wise choices as I purchase, prepare and eat the food that you have provided. May each bite be a small step taken in the direction of divine health and healing in my body, and let every choice I make bring glory to your name. Amen.

What's In a Label? – Chapter Review

- The USFDA's Nutrition Facts label is one way to determine what is in a food product and whether you should purchase or consume it.
- Determine your serving size and how many calories you will be consuming.
- Limit your intake of saturated fats and avoid all trans fats.
- Avoid high levels of cholesterol and sodium, especially important if you have high cholesterol, heart problems, high blood pressure or a history of heart disease.
- Strive for a high-fiber diet.
- Avoid foods high in sugar, which get digested quickly and trigger the release of insulin.
- Check the ingredients list to determine what type of sugar(s) it contains.
- Choose nutrient-rich foods over foods that are nutrient deficient.
- Check the Percentage of Daily Values (or %DV) to determine what percentage of nutrients you will be getting.
- Read through the ingredients listing. Avoid food products filled with chemicals, food dyes and food additives.

Do you make it a habit to check Nutrition Fact labels when purchasing foods? Are you now better equipped to understand food labeling? _____

_____

_____

Do you think that a better understanding of Nutrition Fact labels and ingredient lists will help you make wiser food choices?

_____

Why?_____

_____

_____

Browse through your pantry and look at a few Nutrition Fact labels. Are there any foods that you once considered "healthy" which now seem less beneficial? _____

_____

_____

At the store, compare two different brands of the same food. Which of the two is healthier for your family? _____

_____

_____

What foods are you more committed to avoiding or eliminating from your diet? _____

_____

_____

Make it your habit to buy fewer processed, man-made foods and more organic "God-made" foods. Can you think of any healthy substitutions that can be made for processed foods you currently consume (ie. almonds instead of potato chips, pretzels instead of candy, celery with healthy peanut butter instead of cookies, sparkling water instead of soda)? _____

_____

_____

_____

_____

_____

_____

Notes: _____

_____

_____

_____

_____

_____

_____

_____

The only thing I like better
than talking about food
is eating.

—✺—

JOHN WALTERS

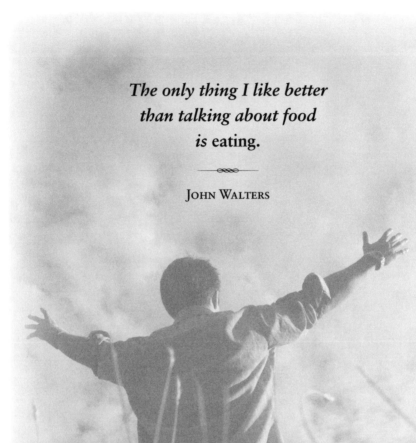

Chapter Seven

God's Top Ten
Constructive Super Foods

TWO-THIRDS OF WHAT WE EAT should be living foods, preferably organic fruits, vegetables and whole grains. It is an established fact that the more fruits and vegetables you eat, the lower your chances of developing heart disease, cancer, and many other health problems. Even adding one serving a day can make a difference!

Many times a diet rich in fruits and vegetables is able to reduce your blood pressure significantly. People who eat more than four servings a day also have significantly lower levels of bad cholesterol. Studies clearly show that fruits and especially vegetables are the best medicine you can take for preventing cancer. Their natural phytonutrients have anti-cancer properties.

Eat your fruits and vegetables raw or steamed, because food in its fresh state retains all its enzymes. Enzymes are the chemical spark plugs in your body that start or speed up chemical processes. There are thousands of enzymes inside you. They take proteins, fats and carbohydrates and structure them to form your body. When you eat fruits and vegetables that still have their enzymes, you boost your body's ability to re-create and protect itself.

Fruits and vegetables should be eaten unpeeled whenever possible because many vitamins and minerals are concentrated in the skin. The outer layer of organic fruits and vegetables should be safe to eat. If you eat non-organic produce, it is imperative that you wash these fruits and vegetables thoroughly to remove as much pesticide residue as possible.

Listed below are ten of God's best, most nutritious foods:[9]

Almonds

Almonds are a great source of calcium, magnesium, phosphorous, copper, protein and anti-inflammatory nutrients. They provide significant amounts of monounsaturated fat, vitamins and phytosterols and are an excellent source of fiber, vitamin E and minerals in general. Nuts are an excellent alternative to snack foods. They are nutritious, provide energy and are very low on the glycemic scale.

Kissing Cousins - walnuts, peanuts, cashews

---

9   You can read more about the foods listed here at www.nutritiondata.com and in Super Health by Craichy.

Apples

Apples are a good source of potassium, phosphorous, fiber, amino acids, phytochemicals, vitamin C and super antioxidants. Many studies indicate that apples decrease the risk of heart disease, cancer and stroke and may lower diabetes risk. Apples also enhance the absorption of other nutrients.

Kissing Cousins – pears

Avocados

Avocados are a great source of mono-unsaturated fatty acids, fiber, magnesium, folate, vitamin E, carotenoids, lutein, vitamin C, vitamin K, vitamin B6, vitamin B12, potassium, zinc, copper, manganese and polyphenol.

Kissing Cousins – asparagus, artichokes, extra virgin olive oil

Beets

Beets are an excellent source of amino acids, vitamin A, vitamin C, magnesium, potassium, fiber, folate and manganese. Beets are known to be very beneficial in helping with liver and gall bladder function.

Kissing Cousins – turnips, carrots, sweet potatoes

Blueberries

Blueberries are a great source of proteins, fiber, antioxidants, lutein, B vitamins, vitamin C, vitamin K, manganese, beta carotene, vitamin E, phosphorous, zinc, copper, magnesium and potassium. Blueberries are a rich source of the antioxidant anthocyanin which gives them their reddish-blue color. They help neutralize the effects of free radical damage in cells.

Kissing Cousins – purple grapes, cranberries, boysenberries, raspberries, strawberries, blackberries and cherries

Broccoli

Broccoli is an excellent food source of vitamins, minerals and proteins, including antioxidants, vitamin C, vitamin A and vitamin K. It also provides significant amounts of fiber, folate, calcium, manganese, magnesium, phosphorous, potassium and selenium. Brought to America by the Italians, broccoli is prized for its taste and nutritional benefits. It has tumor prevention qualities as well as sulfur-containing compounds that have cancer prevention benefits.

Kissing Cousins – brussel sprouts, cabbage, cauliflower, kale

Carrots

Carrots are best known for vitamin A, carotene and eye nutrition. They are a good source of fiber, vitamin C, vitamin B6, vitamin K, pantothenic acid, iron, potassium and copper.

Kissing Cousins – turnips, sweet potatoes, beets

Eggs

Eggs are a great source of protein, vitamin A, vitamin D, pantothenic acid, riboflavin, phosphorous, sodium and selenium. Free-range organic eggs are the best choice.

Kissing Cousins – organic meats such as chicken, beef, turkey, duck and goose eggs

Garlic

One of the oldest cultivated plants in the world, garlic is known for its flavor and anti-viral, anti-inflammatory and anti-biotic properties. It is rich in sulfur-containing compounds and is a good source of calcium, vitamin C, vitamin B6, saponius, phosphorous, potassium, zinc, polyphenols and selenium. Garlic also contains significant amounts of vitamin C, vitamin B6 and manganese and is a diverse source of amino acids.

Kissing Cousins – onions, scallions, leeks

Tomatoes

Tomatoes are a good source of B vitamins, vitamin E, magnesium, folate, phosphorous, copper, amino acids and lutein. They provide high amounts of fiber, vitamin A, vitamin K, vitamin C, potassium and manganese and are a rich source of many antioxidants. Tomatoes are becoming famous for their lycopene content, an antioxidant with cancer prevention properties. They also seem to help the skin become less affected by the harmful rays of the sun.

Kissing Cousins – watermelon, grapefruit, papaya

It is wise to include an ample amount of these foods in your regular diet. God has provided many diverse and nutritious foods for us to enjoy which are bursting with explosive flavors and great health benefits. Food is a blessing from God.[10] Realize that just a few months of eating healthy, nutritious foods will

---

10   "Worship the Lord your God, and his blessing will be on your food and water. I will take away sickness from among you..." Exodus 23:25

result in a healthier, more vibrant life. Building a strong nutritional foundation is one of the keys to "living long and strong for Jesus." By eating the healthiest varieties, especially those free of chemicals, we enhance our chances of living out all of our ordained days.

God has provided many diverse and nutritious foods for us to enjoy.

Thank you, Lord, for creating so many wonderful, delicious foods for me to enjoy. Thank you for providing exactly what my body needs to function at its best. Empower me by your Holy Spirit to make wise decisions about what I feed my body. Strengthen me more and more each day as I continue walking in higher levels of divine health and healing. Amen.

God's Top Ten Constructive Super Foods – In Review

- ♛ TWO-THIRDS OF WHAT YOU EAT SHOULD BE LIVING FOODS, PREFERABLY ORGANIC FRUITS, VEGETABLES AND WHOLE GRAINS.

- ♛ GOD'S TOP TEN CONSTRUCTIVE SUPER FOODS ARE:
  1. ALMONDS
  2. APPLES
  3. AVOCADOS
  4. BEETS
  5. BLUEBERRIES
  6. BROCCOLI
  7. CARROTS
  8. EGGS
  9. GARLIC
  10. TOMATOES

- ♛ HEALTHY FOOD IS A BLESSING FROM GOD.

- ♛ CONSUMING GOD'S TOP TEN CONSTRUCTIVE SUPER FOODS AND ALL OF THEIR "KISSING COUSINS" WILL HELP YOU TO WALK IN DIVINE HEALTH.

How many of the constructive super foods listed above are a part of your regular diet? _____

_____

_____

Were there any constructive super foods that you were surprised to see on the list? _____

_____

_____

Choose two constructive super foods that you can add to your diet each week. _____

_____

_____

If there are any foods listed that you particularly dislike, look through the kissing cousins and find an appropriate substitute.

_____

_____

_____

Ask your friends and family if they have some favorite recipes that use a few of the top ten constructive super foods. _____

_____

_____

Notes: _____

_____

_____

_____

_____

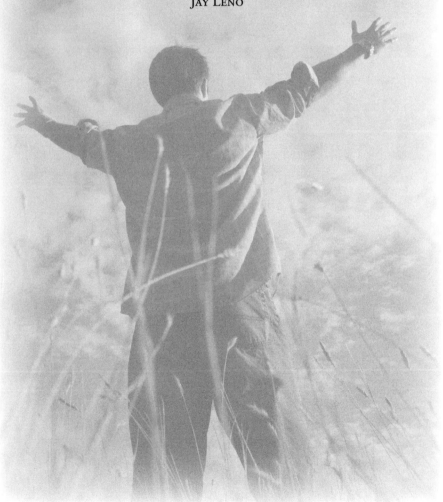

I went into a McDonald's yesterday and said,
"I'd like some fries."

The girl at the counter said,
"Would you like some fries with that?"

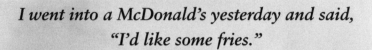

Jay Leno

Chapter Eight

The Top Ten Destructive Foods to Avoid

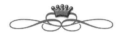

A S WE HAVE DISCUSSED in previous chapters, consuming destructive foods on a regular basis results in cells that are built with second-rate building materials. Tissues and organs become foundationally weak, setting us up for disease over the long term. We literally open the door for the devil to steal our health.

Following is a list of destructive foods that you should avoid or eliminate from your diet:

White Sugar

The biggest problem with white sugar is that it suppresses the immune system. It can also weaken eyesight and speed aging, causing premature wrinkling of the skin. Along with high fructose corn syrup, sugar is the leading cause of diabetes and obesity. It can also cause hyperactivity in children, raise triglycerides in the blood, effect cholesterol levels, contribute to osteoporosis, cancer, hypoglycemia and joint pain.[11]

Sugar is addictive for many people. It raises insulin levels which can lead to high blood pressure, high cholesterol, heart disease, diabetes and weight gain.

The average person consumes their body weight in white refined sugar annually in addition to 20 pounds of high fructose corn syrup.

White Flour

White flour is produced by the heavy processing and bleaching of nutritious wheat germ. The resulting white flour has been robbed of almost all its nutrition and fiber. Instead, opt for high fiber whole wheat bread, spelt or Ezekiel bread.[12] Foods made with white flour, such as white bread and bagels, digest very quickly, causing an insulin response. It is a suspected cause of arthritis, joint pain and inflammation. Read the labels closely and avoid breads that are filled with conditioners, sugar and preservatives.

Trans Fat

Trans fat is most commonly labeled as "partially hydrogenated oil" and is known to raise bad cholesterol, lower good

---

11   You can read more details on sugar's negative impact on your health in my book, Setting Things Straight. Refer to Chapter One, "The Three Worst Foods to Eat and Why."

12   You can read more about the importance of fiber in my book, Setting Things Straight. See the Chapter "How to Lower Your Cholesterol Without Drugs."

cholesterol, cause inflammation in the body and increase the risk of heart disease and cancer.[13] Do not eat anything that contains trans fat oil in it.

Soft Drinks & Sodas (both diet and regular)

Diet sodas are full of chemicals and artificial sweeteners which very likely contribute to dementia and Alzheimer's disease later in life. Regular soda contains an average of 9 teaspoons of white sugar per 12 ounce can. Soda is known to cause kidney stones is a leading contributor to osteoporosis.

It is clear that the consumption of sodas and sweetened drinks is one of the primary causes fueling the worldwide epidemic of obesity and diabetes. If you are struggling with weight issues, be aware that drinking just one can of soda per day can easily cause a 15 pound weight gain over the course of 6 months.

Pork

It's interesting to note that in the Old Testament God forbade the Israelites from eating pork. Pigs eat absolutely any-thing, live, play and constantly dig in their own excrement and have parasites. These are not the kind of nutritional building blocks you want served regularly on your family's table! They are on my list because they were on God's list.

Shellfish

Once again, shellfish are another food group forbidden to the Israelites in the Old Testament. Shellfish include shrimp,

---

13   Trans Fat is discussed in more depth in my book, Setting Things Straight.

lobster, clams, oysters and mussels. All are bottom feeders that too often contain heavy metal toxins such as mercury. Farmed varieties are commonly fed antibiotics and some contain food coloring to improve their appearance. Shellfish can be eaten occasionally but should not be a regular, consistent part of your diet.

French Fries

French fries are the most-consumed vegetable in America. They are void of significant nutrition and are very often deep-fried in trans fat oil, making them a very unhealthy food source. You are better off purchasing the healthier baked varieties from your grocer's freezer section and making them at home.

Commercial Peanut Butter

Most commercial peanut butters are loaded with white sugar, trans fat and salt. Instead, purchase a natural peanut, almond or cashew butter without all the added sugar and trans fat. Remember that trans fat is commonly listed as "partially hydrogenated oil" on food labels.

Milk

While it may surprise you that milk makes this list, it is not nearly as good for you or as good a calcium source as we have been led to believe. In its raw form, milk is very nutritious, but milk that has been pasteurized and homogenized has been highly processed, leaving it with much less nutritional value. Many people suffer from allergies due to milk. Some are intolerant to the lactose sugar that is naturally present in milk (known as "lactose intolerance"). Milk contains a protein that human milk does not contain called "casein." Many experts believe this is the reason many people do not tolerate milk and dairy products well in their diets.

In addition, milk often contains residues of antibiotics, growth hormone, herbicides and pesticides. Milk and related dairy products such as skim and low fat varieties, half and half cream and yogurt are heavily processed. All of this processing can cause inflammation and joint pain in the body and tend to increase bad cholesterol while concurrently lowering good cholesterol. Consider the following comments from leading doctors:

"At least 50% of all children in the United States are allergic to milk, many undiagnosed. Dairy products are the leading cause of food allergy, often revealed by constipation, diarrhea, and fatigue. Many cases of asthma and sinus infections are reported to be relieved and even eliminated by cutting out dairy."[14]

"Milk allergies are very common in children... They are the leading cause of the chronic ear infections that plague up to 40% of all children under the age of six."[15]

---

14   Natural Health, July, 1994, Frank Oski, M.D., Chief of Pediatrics at Johns Hopkins Medical School.

15   Julian Whitaker, M.D., "Health & Healing," October 1998, Volume 8, No. 10.

If you must drink milk, purchase an organic brand to minimize the exposure to hormones, pesticides, herbicides and antibiotic residues.

Doughnuts

Doughnuts often contain 400-500 calories each and are full of sugar, saturated fat, trans fat and calories. As a result they taste great and are fun to eat, but there is a high price to be paid. Truthfully, the healthiest part of the doughnut is actually the hole!

Avoiding destructive foods is just as important as adding the constructive ones into your diet. While avoiding the foods listed above will feel challenging at first, I know you will be pleasantly surprised at how much better you will feel. As your body becomes stronger and healthier, avoiding destructive foods will become easier as you work to maintain your new level of health. Cravings for destructive foods actually decrease over time, and you will find that the temptation to indulge becomes weaker. Each small step you take toward divine health will enable you to live long and strong for Jesus, anticipating and enjoying each day He has ordained for you to live.

> *The healthiest part of the doughnut is actually the hole!*

Thank you, Lord, that you promise to give me wisdom when I ask for it. Help me to make wise choices as I consider what to eat each day. Give me the willpower to say, "No," to foods that are destructive to my body. I give your Holy Spirit permission to bring conviction to my heart when I need it. Please bless my journey to divine health, and thank you that I do not walk this path alone but You are with me each step of the way. May every choice I make bring glory to Your Name. Amen.

The Top Ten Destructive Foods to Avoid – In Review

- ♛ CONSUMING DESTRUCTIVE FOODS ON A REGULAR BASIS RESULTS IN CELLS THAT ARE BUILT WITH SECOND-RATE BUILDING MATERIALS.

- ♛ THE TOP TEN DESTRUCTIVE FOODS TO AVOID ARE:

  1. WHITE SUGAR
  2. WHITE FLOUR
  3. TRANS FAT
  4. SOFT DRINKS & SODAS (BOTH DIET AND REGULAR)
  5. PORK
  6. SHELLFISH
  7. FRENCH FRIES
  8. COMMERCIAL PEANUT BUTTER
  9. MILK
  10. DOUGHNUTS

- ♛ THE LONGER YOU AVOID THESE DESTRUCTIVE FOODS THE LESS YOU WILL TEMPTED BY THEM AND THE BETTER YOU WILL FEEL.

- ♛ AVOIDING DESTRUCTIVE FOODS WILL EMPOWER YOU TO WALK IN DIVINE HEALTH AND HEALING.

How many of the destructive foods listed above are a part of your regular diet? _____

_____

_____

Were there any destructive foods that you were surprised to see on the list? _____

_____

_____

What would you say are the top three destructive foods that need to be removed from your diet? _____

_____

_____

Can you think of a particular time of the day when you are most tempted to consume destructive foods? Is there a constructive food that you could substitute when you are tempted? _____

_____

_____

Choose one or two destructive foods that you can eliminate from your diet each week. _____

_____

_____

Notes: _____

_____

_____

_____

_____

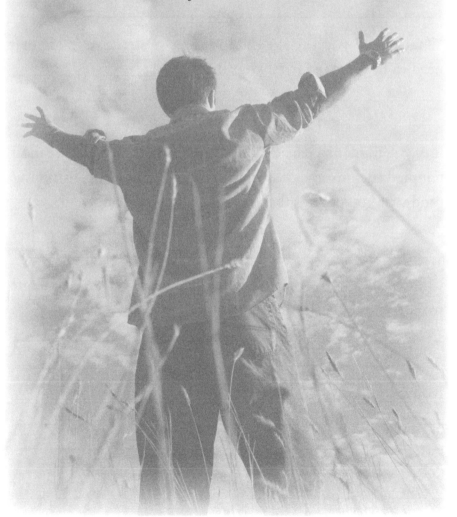

You don't have to cook fancy
or complicated masterpieces —
just good food from fresh ingredients.

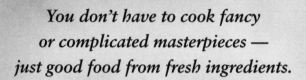

JULIA CHILD

Chapter Nine

Going Organic

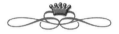

I N ORDER TO FUEL YOUR BODY with the best food available you need to be educated about our food supply. Choosing organic food is sometimes more expensive but is nearly always the best choice for your family. Organic foods are generally described as foods grown or raised without harsh chemicals, fertilizers, pesticides, antibiotics or injected hormones. Attempt to consume organic food whenever it is available.

To avoid confusion, let's start with some simple definitions of words commonly used regarding organic foods:

Organic fruits & vegetables are grown without synthetic pesticides, synthetic fertilizers or sewage sludge and have not been genetically engineered or irradiated.

Organic beef & chicken comes from animals that are raised on 100 percent organic feed and are never given growth hormones, antibiotics or other drugs. In addition, their meat is not irradiated.

Organic milk is from animals that, for at least the past 12 months, are fed 100 percent organic feed and are not given antibiotics or growth hormones.

Organic eggs come from hens that are fed 100 percent organic feed and are not given growth hormones or antibiotics.

"No Antibiotics Added" can appear on a label if the producer can document that the animals were raised without antibiotics.

Poisonous pesticides such as DDT, chlordane and heptachlor were banned from use decades ago, but residues continue to lurk in the soil today.

Increasing public demand for healthier food has made organic choices more widely available than in the past. Organic foods are grown without harmful fertilizers and poisonous pesticides. As a result, foods that are certified organic are healthier and free of cancer-causing chemical residues. You will discover that organic produce is usually smaller and less pretty than its non-organic counterparts. Thankfully, your stomach doesn't see what you put into it and a small organic apple with a few marks is a much wiser choice than a beautiful, shiny one full of harmful chemicals. Organic foods also tend to be a bit more expensive, but we have already determined that you are the crown of God's creation and that divine health is worth the money and the effort! In addition, as demand continues to increase, organic products are becoming much more competitively priced.

Is it really worth the extra money? The answer is a resounding, "Yes!" Organic fruits and vegetables have considerably lower pesticide levels. A study done by the Consumers Union and the Organic Materials Review Institute of Eugene, Oregon reviewed 94,000 samples of 20 different organic crops. Only about one in four contained any pesticide residue. When it *was* detected, the chemicals were usually found in much smaller quantities than in conventionally grown crops. Additionally, it is believed that the pesticides found were simply residue of old pesticide treatment from years past or pesticide drift (chemicals carried in wind and water) from nearby non-organic farms.

> *Organic fruits and vegetables have considerably lower pesticide levels.*

Some foods are naturally resistant to pesticide absorption and chemical residues. The non-profit Environmental Working Group from Washington, D.C., ranked the 43 most commonly consumed fruits and vegetables in order of their pesticide-absorbing tendency. The data used for the ranking included nearly 43,000 analyses conducted by the USDA (U.S. Department of Agriculture) and FDA (United States Food and Drug Administration).

One of the simplest ways to avoid these harmful chemicals is to follow the recommendations of the Environmental Working Group (EWG) by staying away from what they have termed "The Dirty Dozen." By doing so, you can lower your pesticide exposure by nearly 90 percent.

I have included a list of the 12 worst offenders and the 12 fruits and vegetables that had the lowest levels of chemical residues. Number One on the list was peaches, 97 percent of which were contaminated with pesticide residues! The average peach contained three different residues. Soft-skinned fruits and vegetables tended to contain higher residue levels versus those with thicker skins or peels.

The Dirty Dozen

Rank	Fruit or Vegetable	% with Pesticides	% with 2 or more Pesticides
1	Peaches	97%	87%
2	Apples	92%	79%
3	Sweet Bell Peppers	82%	62%
4	Celery	94%	80%
5	Nectarines	97%	85%
6	Strawberries	92%	69%
7	Cherries	91%	76%
8	Pears	87%	47%
9	Grapes[1]	85%	53%
10	Spinach	70%	31%
11	Lettuce	59%	33%
12	Potatoes	81%	18%

[1]Only imported grapes were tested.   Source: Environmental Working Group

Other consistent offenders were carrots, green beans, hot peppers, cucumbers, oranges, tangerines, grapefruit, mushrooms, cauliflower and honeydew melon.

While you would be wise to eliminate pesticides from your family's diet, there are non-organic fruits and vegetables that have significantly lower levels of contamination that may be enjoyed worry-free without the added expense of buying organic varieties. They are listed below as "The Clean Dozen." The Clean Dozen list includes those fruits and vegetables which contain consistently low levels of chemical residues.

The Clean Dozen

Rank	Fruit or Vegetable	% with Pesticides	% with 2 or more Pesticides
1	Onions	0%	0%
2	Avocado	1%	0%
3	Sweet Corn[1]	4%	0%
4	Pineapples	8%	1%
5	Mango	7%	1%
6	Asparagus	7%	1%
7	Sweet Peas[1]	23%	2%
8	Kiwi	15%	3%
9	Bananas	42%	2%
10	Cabbage	18%	5%
11	Broccoli	28%	3%
12	Papaya	24%	5%

[1] Only frozen varieties were tested.   Source: Environmental Working Group

Other fruits and vegetables receiving an honorable mention included blueberries, winter squash, watermelon & tomatoes.

The USDA used to recommend five to seven servings per day of fruits and vegetables. Now it recommends five to thirteen servings a day — almost *double* the previous recommendation! There is no doubt that our bodies need plenty of fresh fruits and vegetables. They are loaded with vitamins, minerals, enzymes, phytonutrients, antioxidants and fiber. God intentionally designed fruits and especially vegetables to be pure fuel and nutrition that would empower your body every day that He ordained for you to live.

Thank you, Lord, for creating the food my body needs to live long and strong for you. Thank you that I have the opportunity to choose foods that are free of pesticides, hormones and antibiotics. Please help me to make wise choices as I purchase, cook and consume the food you've provided for me. I'm so grateful that you walk with me every step of the way on my journey to divine health and healing. Amen.

Going Organic
– In Review

- ❦ ORGANIC FOODS ARE GENERALLY DESCRIBED AS FOODS GROWN OR RAISED WITHOUT HARSH CHEMICALS, FERTILIZERS, PESTICIDES, ANTIBIOTICS OR HORMONES.

- ❦ ATTEMPT TO CONSUME ORGANIC FOOD WHENEVER IT IS AVAILABLE.

- ❦ INCREASING PUBLIC DEMAND FOR HEALTHIER FOOD HAS MADE ORGANIC CHOICES MORE WIDELY AVAILABLE THAN IN THE PAST.

- ❦ AS DEMAND CONTINUES TO INCREASE, ORGANIC PRODUCTS ARE BECOMING MUCH MORE COMPETITIVELY PRICED.

- ❦ BY AVOIDING "THE DIRTY DOZEN," YOU CAN LOWER YOUR PESTICIDE EXPOSURE BY NEARLY 90 PERCENT.

- ❦ THERE ARE NON-ORGANIC FRUITS AND VEGETABLES THAT HAVE SIGNIFICANTLY LOWER LEVELS OF CONTAMINATION THAT MAY BE ENJOYED WORRY-FREE WITHOUT THE ADDED EXPENSE OF BUYING ORGANIC VARIETIES. THEY HAVE BEEN COINED "THE CLEAN DOZEN."

- ❦ THE USDA RECOMMENDS FIVE TO THIRTEEN SERVINGS OF FRUITS AND VEGETABLES A DAY.

- ❦ GOD INTENTIONALLY DESIGNED FRUITS AND ESPECIALLY VEGETABLES TO BE PURE FUEL AND NUTRITION THAT WOULD EMPOWER YOUR BODY AND PROMOTE DIVINE HEALTH AND HEALING.

How many servings of fruits and vegetables do you consume on a typical day? Are you meeting the recommended 5 to 13 servings a day?_____

_____

_____

_____

How can you incorporate more fruits and vegetables into your diet? _____

_____

_____

Do you presently purchase and consume organic foods? ____

_____

_____

If you haven't purchased organic foods because of the cost associated with them, I strongly urge you to revisit the organic section in your local grocery. Many organic foods will fit easily within your budget due to higher demand from consumers.__

_____

_____

_____

Does your family consume organic meat and eggs? This is very important to consider if you have small children, who are especially affected by livestock hormone injections. _____

_____

_____

_____

Choose one or two foods and start replacing your regular purchases with organic ones._____

_____

_____

Notes: _____

_____

_____

_____

_____

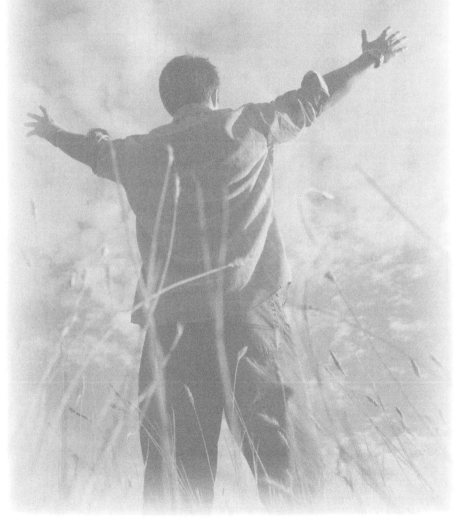

*The best way to detoxify is to
stop putting toxic things into the body
and depend upon its own mechanisms.*

⎯⎯∞⎯⎯

ANDREW WEIL, M.D.

Chapter Ten

Keep Your Machine Clean

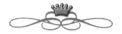

IF YOU ARE LIKE THE AVERAGE AMERICAN, you probably take pretty good care of your car. You visit the car wash when it gets dirty and might even occasionally vacuum out the interior when it gets a bit messy. In addition to keeping it clean on the outside, most of us recognize the importance of maintaining the car's internal integrity as well. Every 3,000 miles the guys at the quick lube place are happy to change the oil and filter for a swipe of your credit card. After all, a car is no cheap machine and it makes sense to take care of our automobiles, inside and out!

I am sad to say that many people take better car of their cars than they do their bodies. While we are generally aware of the external appearance of our body, the function of our insides does not often get much attention until something breaks down and we are suffering with pain or disease.

Many people take better care of their cars than they do their bodies.

—☖—

The facts are sobering. Our bodies are staggering under an enormous load of toxins from the food we eat, the air we breathe and the water supply we drink. The polluted environment exposes us to chemical overload and threatens the health and healing systems God designed within us.

According to the Environmental Working Group, nearly every person in the United States carries more than 100 chemical pollutants, pesticides and toxic metal residues in their bodies. Are you being affected? Yes! Following is a list of symptoms that you may be experiencing as a result of the toxic buildup of chemicals in your body:

- SENSITIVITY TO PERFUMES AND OTHER CHEMICAL ODORS
- PERSISTENT JOIN OR MUSCLE PAIN (IN MULTIPLE AREAS)
- CHRONIC INFECTIONS
- DEPRESSION
- CHRONIC FATIGUE
- CHRONIC HEADACHES WHICH ARE UNRESPONSIVE TO CHIROPRACTIC, MEDICAL OR MASSAGE TREATMENTS

What are the sources of the toxins and chemicals that threaten our health?

Tap water — The municipal tap water we drink is purified with chlorine (which kills bacteria) but is not filtered for chemicals. The use of prescription medications has become so prolific that our newest pollutant in the water is pharmaceuticals. People taking medication pass traces in urine and feces into the sewer system.

In Lake Michigan, researchers found traces of acetaminophen, ibuprofen, birth control hormones and beta blockers from heart medication. In treated water at the Grand Rapids, Michigan, water filtration plant, researchers found the anti-seizure medication carbamazepine. In some parts of the country male fish have developed female ovarian tissue from constant exposure to birth control hormones. While acknowledging that the drugs are measured in parts per trillion (too small to be considered a therapeutic dose in humans), scientists are concerned that no one knows the dangers of lifetime exposure in humans.[16]

A recent study looked at 22 million tap water samples from across the country and detected *over 300 types* of contaminants. Over 140 of these chemicals are unregulated and have no set safety standards. They included 83 agricultural pollutants from pesticides

Tap water samples from across the country detected over 300 types of contaminants.

and fertilizers, 59 linked to waste water treatment and 166 industrial chemicals. Sixteen were linked to immune system damage, 52 to cancer, 41 to reproductive toxicity and 36 to developmental problems.[17]

Processed food — Processed foods are full of chemical additives and food colorings.

---

16   In Touch Health Newsletter, May 2008.

17   Watson, Brenda, N.D. Essential Cleansing for Perfect Health, Clearwater, Florida: Renew Life Press, 2006.

Fish and shellfish — Many varieties of fish and shellfish contain high levels of heavy metals such as mercury.

Prescription and over-the-counter medications — These medicines place a toxic burden on the liver, the main detoxification organ in the body.

Vaccines — In addition to their active ingredients, vaccines contain mercury, aluminum, antifreeze and formaldehyde. (This includes flu vaccines.)

Amalgam dental fillings — As the acid in our saliva slowly degrades fillings, they leach metal and chemicals into our digestive systems.

Toothpastes — Toothpastes contain fluoride, which is highly toxic in large quantities, as well as other chemicals and colorings.

Hair dyes — Hair dyes are full of dangerous chemicals and their ingredients may absorb through the scalp while being applied.

Lotions and cosmetics — Most suntan lotions, body lotions and cosmetics are produced with petroleum-based ingredients which are readily absorbed through the skin. Many mascaras and eyeliners contain lead or coal-based derivatives.

Cigarette smoke, including second-hand smoke — Cigarette smoke contains more than fifty noxious chemicals. Eleven of these are known carcinogens (cancer-causing).

Thankfully, you and I are in control of nearly every one of these potential sources of toxins. The key to keeping your machine clean is to prevent impurities from entering it in the first place. Here are some simple and practical ways to eliminate toxins from your environment and your body:

- ☙ DRINK LOTS OF PURE WATER. CONSIDER INSTALLING A REVERSE OSMOSIS WATER PURIFICATION SYSTEM IN YOUR HOME FOR DRINKING AND COOKING. DRINK HALF YOUR BODY'S WEIGHT IN OUNCES. FOR EXAMPLE, IF YOU WEIGH 150 POUNDS YOU SHOULD STRIVE TO DRINK 75 OUNCES OF PURE WATER DAILY. WATER FLUSHES TOXINS AND WASTE MATERIALS FROM YOUR BODY AND IS ONE OF THE SIMPLEST WAYS TO KEEP YOUR MACHINE CLEAN.

- ☙ INSTALL A CHLORINE FILTER ON YOUR SHOWER TO MINIMIZE BREATHING CHLORINE AND FLUORIDE DIRECTLY INTO YOUR LUNGS THROUGH SHOWER STEAM.

- ☙ AVOID PROCESSED FOODS AND INSTEAD PURCHASE AND SERVE ORGANIC, CONSTRUCTIVE FOODS. THESE FOODS CONTAIN SIGNIFICANTLY LESS LEVELS OF CHEMICALS TOXINS AND POLLUTANTS.

- ☙ INCREASE THE FIBER IN YOUR DIET. FIBER ABSORBS TOXINS IN THE INTESTINAL TRACT AND HELPS EXCRETE THEM MORE READILY FROM YOUR BODY.

- ☙ AVOID FISH AND SHELLFISH THAT ARE KNOWN TO CONTAIN HIGH LEVELS OF MERCURY AND OTHER METALS.

- ☙ MINIMIZE PRESCRIPTION AND OVER-THE-COUNTER MEDICATIONS.

- ☙ UNTIL SAFER VACCINES ARE DEVELOPED, DO NOT EXPOSE YOUR FAMILY TO THE TOXINS CONTAINED IN VACCINATIONS. INSTEAD, CHOOSE TO FIGHT DISEASE NATURALLY WITH THE PRECEPTS OUTLINED IN THIS BOOK.

- ☙ MAKE WISE CHOICES REGARDING DENTAL CARE. WHEN IT IS TIME TO HAVE A FILLING REPLACED, REQUEST A

WHITE OR COMPOSITE FILLING INSTEAD OF A METAL ONE. PURCHASE FLUORIDE-FREE TOOTHPASTE FOR YOUR FAMILY. BE SURE TO WARN YOUR CHILDREN NOT TO SWALLOW TOOTHPASTE.

- BUY COSMETICS THAT ARE FREE FROM PETROLEUM-BASED INGREDIENTS. THERE ARE MANY EXCELLENT NATURAL COSMETICS AVAILABLE SUCH AS ARBONNE, DEMOLOGICA AND OTHERS.

- CHOOSE LOTIONS AND SUNSCREEN THAT ARE MORE NATURAL AND FREE FROM HARSH INGREDIENTS. BECOME AN EXPERT AT LABEL-READING.

- IF YOU SMOKE, MAKE A PLAN TO QUIT AND SURROUND YOURSELF WITH ENCOURAGING PEOPLE WHO WILL PRAY FOR YOU AND HOLD YOU ACCOUNTABLE. AVOID FREQUENTING PLACES THAT ARE FILLED WITH SECOND-HAND SMOKE.

- AVOID BREATHING FUMES FROM CAR AND TRUCK EXHAUST, BEAUTY SALONS, CHEMICAL PLANTS, HOUSEHOLD PRODUCTS, ETC.

- CHOOSE A VIGOROUS EXERCISE THAT YOU ENJOY AND FIND A PARTNER WHO WILL KEEP YOU MOTIVATED. EXERCISE STIMULATES YOUR BLOOD CIRCULATION AND LYMPHATIC SYSTEM. WALKING, RUNNING, BICYCLING, ROWING, SWIMMING, FAST DANCING AND JUMPING ROPE ARE JUST A FEW EXAMPLES OF EXCELLENT FORMS OF AEROBIC EXERCISE THAT WILL HELP YOUR BODY ELIMINATE TOXINS AND KEEP YOU HEALTHY.

These simple ideas will eliminate toxins before they have the opportunity to steal your health; however, there are toxins that are almost unavoidable in our society. What can be done about them?

The best news of all is that God built an automatic detoxification system into your body that is at work even now. He is such an awesome Creator! Your skin, lungs, digestive system, liver, kidneys and lymphatic system are all part of His design to eliminate toxins from your body.

Your skin, of course, is the first physical barrier against toxins you might come into contact with. In addition, skin releases toxins and impurities through perspiration (which is why body odor is unpleasant). Your lungs eliminate toxic waste from the body in the form of carbon dioxide. Toxins that enter the body through the digestive tract are transported to the liver. They are first

> *God built an automatic detoxification system into your body.*

neutralized and are then excreted through the intestines. The liver is constantly working to clean and filter the 100 gallons of blood that flow through it every 24 hours. The kidneys also help purify the bloodstream and eliminate waste products and toxins from the body. Finally, the lymphatic system maintains detoxification of organs, cells and tissues and aids the liver in purifying the bloodstream.

If you are chronically sick or have a disease such as cancer, fibromyalgia, chronic fatigue syndrome or multiple sclerosis you should consider consulting with a natural health care provider. This may include a nutritionist, chiropractor, holistic dentist, massage therapist and colon hydrotherapist. These professionals can assist you in eliminating toxins more aggressively from your body through herbal therapies, colonic therapy, controlled fasting, dieting advice, accountability and lifestyle counseling.

Our world may be full of toxins but *your body does not have to be!* You can make choices today that will help keep your body clean and running smoothly. Each small choice is a step in the direction of divine health and healing.

L ord, thank you for creating in my body the ability to remove dangerous toxins. Please help it to be strong and clean so that I can serve you better. Thank you that you will give me the strength and willpower to make wise choices about what I expose my body to. Protect my body from the harmful effects of toxins that do make their way inside me. May I continually move toward divine health and healing with every choice I make. Amen.

Keep Your Machine Clean
– In Review

- ♛ AMERICANS ARE EXPOSED TO A STAGGERING AMOUNT OF TOXINS.

- ♛ THE SOURCES OF TOXINS INCLUDE TAP WATER, AIR, PROCESSED FOODS, FISH AND SHELLFISH, MEDICATION, VACCINES, DENTAL TREATMENTS AND PRODUCTS, PERSONAL CARE ITEMS AND CIGARETTE SMOKE.

- ♛ THE EASIEST WAY TO ENSURE DETOXIFICATION IS TO AVOID TOXINS IN THE FIRST PLACE.

- ♛ WHEN IT IS IMPOSSIBLE TO AVOID TOXINS, GOD CREATED AN AUTOMATIC DETOXIFICATION SYSTEM IN OUR BODIES TO DEAL WITH THEM.

Be honest with yourself. Do you take better care of your car than you do your body? _____

_____

_____

Are you suffering from any of the symptoms that indicate toxicity? _____

_____

_____

_____

What toxins are you frequently exposed to? _____

_____

_____

_____

What choices can you make to limit your exposure to toxins?

_____

_____

_____

Notes: _____

_____

_____

_____

_____

_____

_____

_____

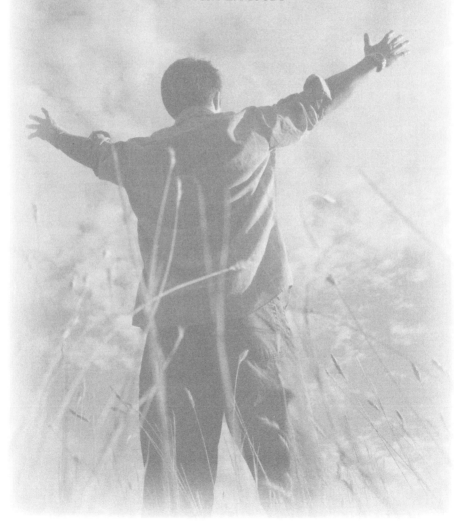

God doesn't seek for golden vessels,
and does not ask for silver ones,
but He must have clean ones.

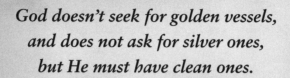

DWIGHT L. MOODY

Chapter Eleven

Closing the Door on Cancer

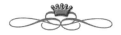

CANCER IS A HORRIBLE DISEASE that claims the lives of far too many Christians. As the second leading cause of death in the United States, cancer strikes the body in no less than 100 different forms. According to the American Cancer Society, half of all men and one third of all women in our country will develop the disease during their lifetime.

What exactly is cancer? To understand how it forms, let's quickly revisit the normal function of a cell. Cells grow, divide and die in an orderly fashion. This constant cell death and regeneration is an amazing part of God's design in our bodies. One cell dies and another one exactly the same in structure and function is created to take its place. Cells reproduce themselves using DNA, the genetic blueprint of the cell that governs cell properties and function. Occasionally DNA becomes damaged, but a healthy body has the ability to repair the DNA without any impact on cell reproduction.

This leads us to the circumstances that open the door for cancer to develop. If DNA becomes damaged and a person's body isn't healthy enough to fix it, that single damaged cell will reproduce itself using a faulty blueprint. The result is more deformed cells, who themselves go on to reproduce. The end result is a group or mass of deformed cells — a tumor.

When a person's immune system is strong cancer cells will normally be destroyed.

God created a backup plan. When a person's immune system is strong, any cancer cells that do develop will normally be destroyed, preventing them from multiplying and forming tumors. Unfortunately, many times the problem goes unrecognized by the body until the cancer has progressed too far and overwhelms the body's defenses. No matter what type of cancer is involved, most all start in this manner due to DNA damage which the body is unable to repair. We will discuss the actual cause of this damage shortly.

Some cancers, like leukemia, involve free-floating blood cells and do not form tumors. Some forms of cancer start in one part of the body and spread to other parts. This process is called "metastasis." Different types of cancer behave very differently from one another. They grow at different rates, some spread while others do not, and some forms are more easily treated than others.

Common Cancer Symptoms

The presence of one or more of these symptoms does not necessarily mean that you have cancer but definitely merits seeing a physician for evaluation and further testing.

- ❦ UNEXPLAINED WEIGHT LOSS

- ❦ LASTING FEVER WITHOUT A KNOWN CAUSE

- ❦ UNEXPLAINED FATIGUE

- ❦ UNRELENTING PAIN, ESPECIALLY IN THE HEAD, CHEST OR ABDOMEN

- ❦ CHANGE IN BLADDER AND/OR BOWEL HABITS

- ❦ THICKENING OR LUMPS IN THE BODY

- ❦ UNUSUAL BLEEDING OR DISCHARGES

- ❦ CHANGES OF COLOR AND/OR SIZE IN MOLES

- ❦ CHRONIC COUGH AND/OR HOARSENESS

- ❦ COUGHING UP BLOOD

- ❦ SORES THAT DO NOT HEAL

- ❦ CHRONIC INDIGESTION AND/OR DIFFICULTY SWALLOWING

- ❦ CHRONIC HEAD PAIN OR BLURRED VISION

Traditional Cancer Treatment

The four most common methods of traditional or conventional cancer treatment are:

- ❦ SURGERY TO REMOVE THE TUMOR AND AFFECTED TISSUES

- ❦ RADIATION TO KILL CANCEROUS CELLS

- ❦ CHEMOTHERAPY TO KILL CANCEROUS CELLS

♛ DRUG THERAPIES TO SUPPRESS CANCER GROWTH

These methods are often used concurrently in treatment.

Alternative Cancer Therapies

Alternative, non-traditional therapies are primarily used to enhance the body's own natural healing and recuperative abilities. Common forms of natural health care designed to assist natural healing are:

♛ CHIROPRACTIC CARE

♛ DIET AND NUTRITION

♛ HERBS, VITAMINS AND MINERALS

♛ MASSAGE THERAPY, REFLEXOLOGY

♛ ACUPUNCTURE, BIOFEEDBACK

♛ HOMEOPATHY

♛ BODY DETOXIFICATION, COLON HYDROTHERAPY

♛ HYPERBARIC OXYGEN THERAPY

♛ PRAYER, MEDITATION, VISUALIZATION

So what actually causes cancer? What causes the DNA damage in the first place? Why are some people's bodies able to repair damaged DNA without any problems, while others cannot and end up facing a difficult battle for health and life? Let's discuss some known causes of DNA damage. If we understand what causes the damage, we are well on our way to preventing it in the first place.

Known Causes of DNA Damage

Tobacco products – It has been proven for years that smoking greatly increases the risk of lung cancer as well as heart disease. Chewing tobacco increases the risk of developing cancer of the mouth, tongue and throat. It is estimated that 50 percent of all cancer is directly or indirectly linked to tobacco use. Tobacco smoke contains over 50 toxic chemicals including 11 known carcinogens. It is clear that tobacco use, including chewing tobacco, cigars, pipes and cigarettes, damages cell DNA.

> ❦ BREATHING SECONDHAND SMOKE FOR EVEN A BRIEF TIME CAN HAVE IMMEDIATE ADVERSE EFFECTS ON THE CARDIOVASCULAR SYSTEM, INTERFERING WITH NORMAL FUNCTION OF THE HEART, LUNGS AND BLOOD VESSELS.

> ❦ NON-SMOKERS WHO ARE EXPOSED TO SECONDHAND SMOKE AT HOME OR AT WORK ARE 20-30 PERCENT MORE LIKELY TO DEVELOP LUNG CANCER AND HEART DISEASE.

The five worst chemicals found in tobacco smoke are:

1. *Arsenic* – *the notorious "poison of choice" used by criminals in the good old days*

2. *Cyanide* – *the chemical most often used in gas chambers*

3. *Ammonia* – *causes nicotine to be more freely absorbed*

4. *Cadmium* – *an ingredient in batteries, paints and pigments*

5. *Nicotine* – *the prime addictive agent of tobacco*

Alcohol – Alcohol use increases the risk of developing cancer of the mouth, throat and digestive tract and is a primary cause of cancer of the liver. The risk is compounded when a person smokes *and* drinks. There are also increased rates of cancer of the breast, colon and liver associated with excessive alcohol consumption.

Heavy Sun Exposure – Skin cancer is one of the most common forms of DNA damage and results from exposure to UV radiation. Sun exposure is healthy in moderate amounts. It appears that strong, intense exposure over years and multiple, extreme sunburns are the most damaging.

Radiation Exposure – High levels of radiation exposure are known to cause cancer, such as radioactive fallout from nuclear weapons testing and nuclear disasters such as occurred at Chernobyl. Excessive use of certain medical procedures, especially x-rays, has been connected to higher cancer rates.[18]

Sexual Behaviors – People who have sex with multiple partners are more prone to develop penile, labial, oral, uterine and anal cancer. Increased cervical cancer rates in women are thought to be connected to contraction of the Human Papilloma Virus (HPV).

Environmental Carcinogens – The American Cancer Society states that exposure to environmental factors is the cause of 75 percent of all cancers.[19] Consistent exposure to fumes, breathing of benzenes from automobile exhaust and incinerators, pesticides, herbicides and fertilizers are all known to increase the risk of developing cancer.

---

18   Typical medical and dental x-rays are considered safe.

19   Alcohol and tobacco use are included in the list of environmental factors.

Obesity – A study done in Sweden by the Karolinska Institute tracked 28,129 obese patients from 1965 through 1993. Compared to non-obese people, they were more likely to develop cancer of the small intestine, larynx, colon, gall bladder, cervix, uterus, ovary, brain, connective tissues and lymph glands. A person is considered obese if they are 20 percent over their ideal weight. (For example, if your ideal weight is 170 pounds, you are considered obese if you are 34 pounds overweight.) Morbid obesity is defined as being 100 pounds overweight.

High Estrogen Levels – Birth control pills and estrogen-based hormone medications such as those used to treat menopausal symptoms are known to increase the risk of developing breast, uterine and ovarian cancers.

Stress & Emotional Factors – Excessive emotional fatigue as a result of unrelenting stress, anxiety, constant fear, ceaseless worry and prolonged unforgiveness are other factors that likely increase the risk of cancer development.

Genetics – According to the American Cancer Society, only five to ten percent of all cancer is genetically caused. It is true that you are more likely to develop certain types of cancer if they run in your family; however, as Christians we can and should trust God to prevent cancer from ever attacking our bodies.

Choices regarding healthy lifestyles, dietary habits, exercise routines, etc., play an incredibly large role in whether we will ever personally face battling cancer. While we trust God for His protection and blessing we must also be willing to do our part in preventing cancer from ever developing in our own bodies.

> *We must be willing to do our part in preventing cancer.*
> —⚜—

While all of the known causes of cancer can seem somewhat daunting, we have so much control over avoiding it. Our wonderful Creator built into each and every person's body the amazing ability to adapt to his or her environment. For example, not all people living in New York City develop cancer even though they are consistently exposed to higher levels of stress, noise and pollution than their counterparts in rural America. In the same way, not all smokers develop lung cancer, nor do all those who drink alcohol develop liver cancer.

DNA damage and the resulting abnormal cell development appear to occur in everyone's body; however, the majority of the time it is repairable by the body. Cancer only develops when the body is unable to repair or heal itself.

Finding a Cure is Not the Answer

Because cancer is likely caused by tens of thousands of physical and environmental factors, finding a cure is not a time or cost-productive method for defeating this horrible disease. Billions upon billions of dollars have been spent since U.S. President Richard Nixon waged the "war on cancer" in the 1970's, but cancer remains the number two killer almost four decades later.

Because it will take more years than you and I have to live for scientists and researchers to determine all the causes, treatments and cures, it becomes *our* responsibility to stop cancer at our own front door!

Matthew 12:29 says, "How can anyone enter a strong man's house and carry off his possessions unless he first ties up the strong man? Then he can rob his house."

You are the strong man in control of your own house as long as you are making decisions that lead to divine health. Do not allow anyone to come along, tie you up and ruin your health!

> *You are the strong man in control of your own house.*

I hope you are feeling empowered and excited to start making wiser choices that will keep cancer far away from your life and your family. In the next chapter we'll discuss the two main ways to stop cancer from stealing your health. Choose today to joyfully live out all of the days God has ordained for you.

Thank you, Lord, that cancer is not an inevitable disease and that I don't have to live in fear and dread of it. Thank you for giving me the knowledge and wisdom to make wise choices. Fill me with your Holy Spirit and give me courage to make the practical changes that will lead to divine health in my body, soul and spirit. I trust You to protect my health as we co-labor to bring glory to Your Name. Amen.

Closing the Door on Cancer
– In Review

- ⚜ ACCORDING TO THE AMERICAN CANCER SOCIETY, HALF OF ALL MEN AND ONE THIRD OF ALL WOMEN IN OUR COUNTRY WILL DEVELOP THE DISEASE DURING THEIR LIFETIME.

- ⚜ CELLS REPRODUCE THEMSELVES USING DNA, THE GENETIC BLUEPRINT OF THE CELL THAT GOVERNS CELL PROPERTIES AND FUNCTION. DNA OFTEN BECOMES DAMAGED BUT A HEALTHY BODY HAS THE ABILITY TO REPAIR ITSELF WITHOUT ANY IMPACT ON CELL REPRODUCTION.

- ⚜ IF DNA BECOMES DAMAGED AND A PERSON'S BODY ISN'T HEALTHY ENOUGH TO FIX IT, THAT SINGLE DAMAGED CELL WILL REPRODUCE USING A FAULTY BLUEPRINT. THE RESULT IS MORE DEFORMED CELLS, WHO THEMSELVES GO ON TO REPRODUCE. THE END RESULT IS A GROUP OR MASS OF DEFORMED CELLS — A TUMOR.

- ⚜ CANCER ONLY DEVELOPS WHEN THE BODY IS UNABLE TO REPAIR OR HEAL ITSELF.

- ⚜ IF YOU ARE EXHIBITING ANY OF THE COMMON SYMPTOMS OF CANCER LISTED IN THE CHAPTER, YOU SHOULD SEE YOUR DOCTOR.

- ⚜ COMMON MEDICAL CANCER TREATMENTS INCLUDE SURGERY, CHEMOTHERAPY, RADIATION AND DRUGS.

- ⚜ THERE ARE MANY ALTERNATIVE CANCER TREATMENTS AVAILABLE.

♛ KNOWN CAUSES OF DNA DAMAGE AND CANCER ARE:

1. TOBACCO PRODUCTS

2. ALCOHOL

3. HEAVY SUN EXPOSURE

4. RADIATION EXPOSURE

5. SEXUAL BEHAVIORS

6. ENVIRONMENTAL CARCINOGENS

7. OBESITY

8. HIGH ESTROGEN LEVELS

9. STRESS AND EMOTIONAL FACTORS

10. GENETICS

♛ FINDING A CURE IS NOT A TIME OR COST-PRODUCTIVE METHOD OF DEFEATING THIS HORRIBLE DISEASE.

♛ IT IS OUR RESPONSIBILITY TO KEEP CANCER FROM ATTACKING OUR BODIES.

How many people do you know personally who have been diagnosed with cancer? _____

_____

_____

_____

How many people do you know personally who have died from cancer? _____

_____

_____

_____

Have you just assumed that cancer is an inevitable part of life? Do you feel differently after reading this chapter? _____

_____

_____

_____

How many of the known causes of DNA damage are you regularly exposed to? _____

_____

_____

_____

What changes can you make to limit the DNA damage in your body? _____

_____

_____

_____

_____

What can you do to enhance your own body's ability to heal
itself?_____

_____

_____

_____

Choose two changes that you can make today so that cancer
will not be invited to take up residence within your body. ___

_____

_____

_____

Notes: _____

_____

_____

_____

_____

_____

_____

Disease and ill health are caused largely by damage at the molecular and cellular level, yet today's surgical tools are too large to deal with that kind of problem.

RALPH MERKLE

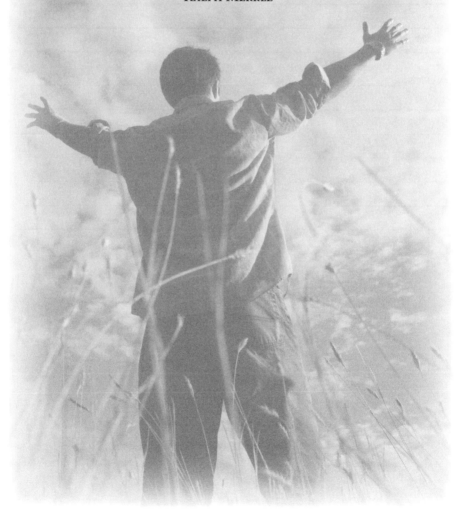

Chapter Twelve

Cancer-Proofing Your Life

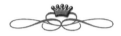

NOW THAT WE HAVE DISCUSSED what cancer is, how it occurs, the symptoms that accompany it, methods of treatment and risk factors, let us focus our attention on the practical steps you can take to avoid facing this terrible disease.

There are two main keys to cancer-proofing your life:

1. *Minimize your exposure to cancer-causing chemicals and behaviors that increase the risk of developing cancer.*

2. *Enhance yo.ur body's God-given ability to heal itself by pursuing divine health.*

Each of these battlegrounds offers us the opportunity to defeat cancer in many simple and practical ways. We will discuss each in turn.

KEY #1   MINIMIZE YOUR EXPOSURE TO CANCER-CAUSING
CHEMICALS AND BEHAVIORS THAT INCREASE THE RISK
OF DEVELOPING CANCER.

By minimizing toxic chemicals in our daily lives and avoiding behaviors which increase our risk, we can drastically lower the possibility of ever receiving a dreadful cancer diagnosis.

We discussed some known causes of increased cancer risk in the last chapter, so avoiding them becomes a simple way of keeping cancer out of our lives.

1. *Avoid using tobacco-related products and breathing other's second-hand smoke. This may mean avoiding bars and restaurants that are thick with smoke.*

2. *Avoid excessive alcohol use.*

3. *Avoid excessive sun exposure. Although sun exposure is healthy in moderate amounts, avoid intense sun exposure and sunburns.20*

4. *Avoid radiation exposure. Avoid overuse of medical procedures which use high levels of x-ray radiation such as CT scans. Typical medical, dental and chiropractic x-rays are considered safe.*

5. *Make wise, godly choices regarding sexual behavior. Having sex with multiple or same-sex partners opens a wide door of opportunity for disease. Monogamous sex, however, provides protection from sexually transmitted diseases and all of the wonderful benefits of a loving, committed marriage.*

---

20   Most sunscreens include high amounts of petroleum-based chemicals. A number of healthier, less chemically intense versions are available.

6. *Minimize your exposure to environmental carcinogens.*

- Minimize dry cleaning services to avoid exposure to chemicals used in the cleaning process.

- Use as little chlorine bleach and detergent as possible when washing your family's clothes.

- Use a chlorine filter on your showerhead. When you breathe steam from chlorinated water you ingest chlorine and fluoride directly into your lungs.[21]

- Avoid nail and hair salons with heavy fumes. Instead, use more natural methods of nail and hair care in your own home.

- Limit mercury exposure. Find a mercury-free dentist (more commonly called a "holistic" dentist) who uses only mercury-free fillings.

- Minimize or eliminate flu shots and vaccines, which commonly contain high levels of mercury, aluminum and formaldehyde as preservatives.

- Refrain from breathing automobile and truck fumes which contain benzenes and many other toxic chemicals. If possible, choose a home located away from busy streets and interstates to avoid breathing heavy petrochemical fumes on a consistent basis.

- Avoid living downwind from power and manufacturing plants.

---

21   My mother died of lung cancer and never smoked, but for several decades she showered in a very confined bathroom with poor ventilation. She was also exposed to secondhand smoke in her family home. I believe both of those factors were responsible for her cancer.

– Drink and cook with purified water. Ideally, install a reverse osmosis water purification system under your kitchen sink. It is fine to bath in regular tap water, but I don't recommend drinking it on a continual basis. Ground water, in too many areas, is also contaminated with nitrates from farm run-off, industrial compounds, pesticides and herbicides.[22]

– Avoid petroleum-based cosmetics and lotions. Many healthier, plant-based, less toxic varieties of personal care items are available including deodorants, cosmetics, lotions, toothpastes, etc. Remember that *divine health is worth the extra cost and the extra effort!*

– Avoid processed food. Foods packaged in cans and boxes are generally full of chemical additives, enhancers and dyes. Consider this as you purchase drinks, too.

– Avoid soft drinks and sports drinks which contain huge amounts of food coloring, chemical additives, white sugar and/or artificial sweeteners. If you can't pronounce it – don't eat it!

– Avoid preserved meats like cured hams, hot dogs, bacon and salami. They are full of nitrates, additives and preservatives.

7. *Maintain a healthy weight. Avoid obesity. We will focus more on a healthy diet in our discussion of pursuing divine health below.*

---

22   Equally frightening is a new health concern regarding our water supplies. Recently, water tested in Grand Rapids, Michigan, was found to be contaminated with prescription medicine residue from psychotropic drugs used to treat depression, anxiety and mental disorders. Just more incentive to insist on clean, pure drinking water!

8. *Normalize estrogen levels. Use caution when deciding to use estrogen-raising medications and birth control pills. Opt for more natural choices to balance hormone levels and prevent conception.*

9. *Minimize stress and emotional factors. Stress is a known health destroyer. There is little doubt that long-term intense stress opens the door to cancer. Getting adequate sleep, exercising, taking vacations and trusting God more are all ways to lower your stress. We will consider this topic in much greater depth in an upcoming chapter.*

KEY #2 ENHANCE YOUR BODY'S GOD-GIVEN ABILITY TO HEAL ITSELF BY PURSUING DIVINE HEALTH.

Visit any local gym and you will find folks working out for any number of reasons. Some are anticipating getting into a bathing suit, a wedding gown or a prom dress in the near future. Others covet a set of "six pack abs" or are attempting to lose weight. But by far, the best reason to pursue divine health is the awareness that God has a plan for your days and that disease can impede the awesome life He intended for you to live.

1. *Get your spine checked for subluxations.*

Subluxation is a medical term for a spinal bone (vertebra) that becomes misaligned. Misalignment is usually caused by trauma, body impact, slips, falls and stress. Subluxations adversely affect the function of your nerve system.

Between 1986 and 1988, Dr. Ronald Pero, an internationally respected cancer researcher, was the principal investigator in the Chiropractic Research Project in Sweden, a study comparing people who had cancer to their healthy counterparts.[23] This was one of the first studies linking DNA damage to cancer and the results were groundbreaking. Pero discovered that healthy people had a *200 percent greater ability to heal their DNA* when it became damaged than those who developed cancer.[24]

What was even more astounding was this: chiropractic patients involved in the study had a 200 percent greater capacity to repair their DNA than even the "healthy" population.[25]

According to this research, maintaining healthy alignment in your spine makes your body as much as 400 percent better able to repair DNA damage and prevent cancer as a result.

In a more recent study, researchers discovered that patients receiving chiropractic care have higher levels of the blood chemicals known as 'thiols.' These chemicals have been shown to be associated with more effective DNA repair in the body.[26]

See your chiropractor on a regular basis. Chiropractic appears to be one of our greatest allies in staying healthy and cancer-free!

23   A Mother's Touch. Retrieved March 22, 2009. http://experienceamotherstouch.com/LongTermBenfits.html.

24   Pero R. "Medical Researcher Excited By CBSRF Project Results." The Chiropractic Journal, August 1989; 32.

25   The chiropractic patients tested received chiropractic care on at least a monthly basis for at least a five-year period of time.

26   Journal of Vertebral Subluxation Research, February 2005

2. *Clean up your diet.*

- **Eat more fresh fruit and fresh vegetables.** They contain many cancer-fighting nutrients and antioxidants. Include mixed green salads in your diet.[27] Avoid skinning or peeling vegetables and fruits since the skin contains significant nutrients and antioxidants.

- **Eat organic fruits and vegetables** to minimize pesticide exposure.

- **Substitute frozen fruits and vegetables** if fresh varieties are not available.

- **Lightly steam or eat vegetables raw.** Overcooking kills important enzymes and vitamins and softens fiber content.

- **Drink purified water.**

- **If you choose to consume milk, insist on organic milk.**

- **Eat organic meats** whenever possible.

- **Use natural sweeteners** like Stevia (an herbal sweetener), agave nectar or honey instead of white refined sugar.

- **Make healthy beverage choices,** including purified water, herbal teas, juice and unsweetened carbonated water drinks such as Perrier, San Pelligreno and LaCroix.

- **Aim for a high fiber diet.** Take a fiber supplement if you do not eat enough nuts, fruits and vegetables. Most

---

27   Avoid iceberg lettuce, which has limited nutritional benefits.

Americans only get 25 percent of required fiber in their diets. Fiber is particularly needed when chronic constipation or a family history of colon cancer is prevalent.

- **Take "whole food" nutritional supplements.** Whole food supplements are all-natural versus synthetic, man-made vitamins. They are generally made from organic ingredients which are more easily absorbed and utilized by the body. My observation is that most vitamin supplements sold in drug stores, grocery stores and large chain stores are synthetic. Most licensed natural health care providers can provide you with whole food, natural, nutritional supplements specific to your particular health needs.

  Generally speaking, all adults should take these daily:

  a. **An all-natural multivitamin and mineral supplement**

  b. **Fish oil or flax oil** – take one tablespoon per hundred pounds of body weight daily. This provides important Omega 3 essential fatty acids known to promote heart health, lower cholesterol, improve mental acuity, hormone balance and reduce joint pain and inflammation.

  c. **Antioxidants** – Many good antioxidant supplements are available. Ask your local health food store or natural health care provider for a specific recommendation. Most antioxidant supplements include a combination of vitamins A,B,C,D and E, the mineral selenium, green tea, turmeric, grapefruit seed extracts, grape seed and pine bark extracts, phytonutrients and CoQ10 to name a few.[28]

3. Get 7-8 hours of sleep per night.

Rest promotes healing. Getting too little sleep lowers immune resistance, particularly when it occurs consistently.

4. Get regular exercise.

Exercise strengthens tissue resistance, increases heart rate and blood flow, intensifies oxygen and nutrient flow to body tissues, helps brain acuity and strengthens immune function and bone strength.

5. Breastfeed.

Breastfeeding has been proven to strengthen immunity in children and provides a strong foundation for lifelong immunity.

6. Get regular cancer screening.

I am not a fan of all medical screening tests, but I do strongly recommend self breast exams, colonoscopy and prostate exams.

7. Guide and guard your thoughts.

Our thoughts are powerful and can make us sick or well. You may have heard the saying, "Perception is reality." Even if your belief is not accurate, the thoughts you dwell on too often tend to become a reality in your life if you think them consistently enough. Guide your thoughts

---

28   Foods supplements are more thoroughly discussed in my book <u>Setting Things Straight</u>. See the chapter entitled "Vitamin Supplements... Where Do I Begin?"

in a positive, life-giving direction and refuse to meditate on negative and worrisome ideas.[29]

8. *Watch your words.*

Words have power much as thoughts do and create our reality.[30] Do not constantly dwell on and speak about sickness. Do not complain about how bad you are feeling. Do not personalize your health challenges by referring to them as "my headache," "my MS," etc. Instead, choose positive words of encouragement and good health and believe God's promises for your best health and life.

9. *Maintain a positive mental attitude.*

In nearly 30 years as a natural health care expert I have worked with many patients diagnosed with cancer. Those who survive *always* have a positive outlook on life. If a positive mental attitude can bring victory over a daunting disease like cancer, it can certainly help you maintain a fuller and more vibrant life.

10. *Forgiveness.*

Forgive others even when they do not deserve it. Unforgiveness causes bitterness and anger which often lead to cancer of the spirit as well as physical cancer and other debilitating illnesses.

Avoiding environmental toxins and behaviors that lead to increased cancer risks usually involves sweeping, long-term decisions. The choices leading to divine health are a

---

29   "Finally, brothers and sisters, whatever is true, whatever is noble, whatever is right, whatever is pure, whatever is lovely, whatever is admirable—if anything is excellent or praiseworthy—think about such things." Philippians 4:8

30   "The tongue has the power of life and death, and those who love it will eat its fruit." Proverbs 18:21

bit trickier as we confront them time after time each day. As we battle cancer on these two important fronts, however, God empowers us to slam the door on this dreadful disease and its impact on our lives and families. I encourage you to choose at least one or two of these ideas to put into practice each week. Little by little you can close the door on cancer and enjoy the benefits of walking in divine health!

Thank you, Lord, that I don't have to live as a victim of whatever disease might try to come my way. Thank you that you created my body to walk in divine health and healing and that your Spirit will give me the courage to make the necessary choices that will close the door on cancer in my life. Bring to my mind those things that you want to change and give me the power to change them. Help me to live long and strong for you each day. Amen.

Cancer-Proofing Your Life
– In Review

- ♛ THERE ARE TWO MAIN KEYS TO CANCER-PROOFING YOUR LIFE:

    1. MINIMIZE YOUR EXPOSURE TO CANCER-CAUSING CHEMICALS AND BEHAVIORS THAT INCREASE THE RISK OF DEVELOPING CANCER.

    2. ENHANCE YOUR BODY'S GOD-GIVEN ABILITY TO HEAL ITSELF BY PURSUING DIVINE HEALTH.

- ♛ BY MINIMIZING TOXIC CHEMICALS IN OUR DAILY LIVES AND AVOIDING BEHAVIORS WHICH INCREASE OUR RISK, WE CAN DRASTICALLY LOWER THE POSSIBILITY OF EVER RECEIVING A DREADFUL CANCER DIAGNOSIS.

- ♛ PURSUING DIVINE HEALTH TO COMBAT CANCER INCLUDES THESE PRACTICAL STEPS:

    1. GET YOUR SPINE CHECKED FOR SUBLUXATIONS.

    2. CLEAN UP YOUR DIET.

    3. GET 7-8 HOURS OF SLEEP PER NIGHT.

    4. GET REGULAR EXERCISE.

    5. BREASTFEED.

    6. GET REGULAR CANCER SCREENING.

    7. GUIDE AND GUARD YOUR THOUGHTS.

    8. WATCH YOUR WORDS.

    9. MAINTAIN A POSITIVE MENTAL ATTITUDE.

    10. FORGIVENESS.

- ♛ GOD HAS EMPOWERED US TO SLAM THE DOOR ON CANCER AND ITS IMPACT ON OUR LIVES AND FAMILIES.

After reading this chapter, do you recognize situations in your life where you are continually exposed to cancer-causing chemicals? _____

_____

_____

Are you presently engaging in a lifestyle and/or behavior that is known to increase the incidence of cancer?_____

_____

_____

_____

Are the foods you eat generally out of a box or a can or are they nutritious "live" foods? _____

_____

Do you suffer from chronic stress?_____

_____

Were you aware of the strong correlation between chiropractic care and reduced cancer risk? Are you under regular chiropractic care? _____

_____

_____

_____

If you do not already take them, find good quality, whole food natural supplements. (Take a multivitamin, mineral, fish oil or flax oil and antioxidant supplement daily.) _____

_____

_____

Do you faithfully get the cancer screenings that are recommended for your age group? _____

_____

_____

_____

Lastly, are you firmly convinced and encouraged that cancer is *not* imminent in the lives of believers? _____

_____

_____

Notes: _____

_____

_____

_____

_____

_____

_____

_____

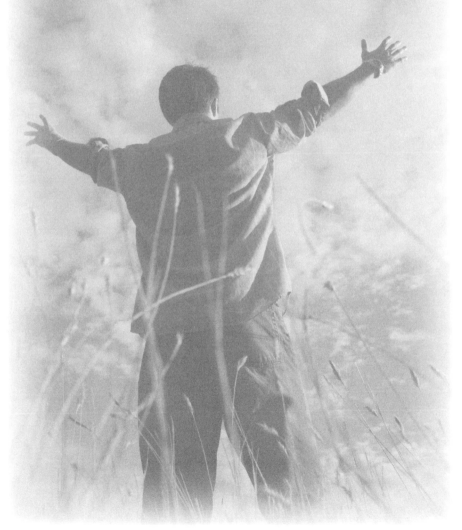

Every human being is the author
of his own health or disease.

———∞∞∞———

BUDDHA

Chapter Thirteen

The Top Ten Killers

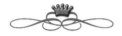

W ALKING EACH DAY IN DIVINE HEALTH means living a joyful, disease-free life. It is my passionate desire to see people – especially Christians – experience the physical, emotional and spiritual health and wholeness that God intended for each one of us. Unfortunately, many are succumbing to sickness and disease.

What does the average American die of today? I call them "The Top Ten Killers" and they claim the lives of 8 out of every 10 people prematurely.

The Top Ten Killers
In the United Sates

Rank	Cause of Death	Deaths per Year
1	Heart Disease	652,486
2	Cancer	553,888
3	Stroke	150,074
4	Lung Diseases[1]	121,987
5	Unintentional Injury[2]	112,012
6	Diabetes	73,138
7	Alzheimer's	65,965
8	Flu and Pneumonia	59,664
9	Kidney Disease	42,480
10	Septicemia/Severe Infections	33,373

Source: U.S. National Center for Health Statistics, 2007

1   Included are chronic obstructive pulmonary disease (COPD), chronic bronchitis, emphysema and asthma.

2   Included are car accidents, drowning, poisoning and other unintentional deaths.

Heart disease and cancer comprise 50 percent of all deaths in the United States. Nearly 8 out of 10 deaths (78 percent) are caused by 1 of the top 10. The four major race groups (European Americans, African Americans, Native Americans and Asian Americans) share 7 of the 10 leading causes of death. Hispanic Americans have 6 of the 10 in common.

Adverse Drug Reactions Leading to Death

It is very interesting to note that deaths from adverse reactions to prescription medications are not included in any

Cause of Death listings from either the U.S. Center for Health Statistics, the World Health Organization or the Center for Disease Control. This is a controversial topic considering that is a commonly understood fact that a minimum of 108,000 people die every year inside U.S. hospitals from reactions to *properly prescribed* FDA-approved prescription medications.

Some estimates of deaths caused by adverse drug reactions range as high as 500,000, increasing its ranking to the second leading killer. Statistical reporting for adverse drug events is poor. Most statistics consider in-hospital deaths only and fail to include deaths from the same that occur in nursing homes or at home. Altogether, these rates would potentially push the ranking to first place.

In ten years' time our nation lost 57,000 Americans in the Vietnam War, and this tragedy continues to stir up emotions even today. It is amazing that there is not a loud outcry as *at least twice that number* dies *every year* due to adverse drug reactions!

Death Due to Doctors and Medical Procedures

An analysis reported in the British Medical Journal concluded that the negative effects of healthcare as practiced in America precipitate 116 million extra visits to the doctor, 77 million additional prescriptions, 17 million more emergency room visits, 8 million more hospitalizations and 199,000 additional deaths — at a cost of 77 billion dollars![31]

---

31   Epidemiology & Medical Error, BMJ, 2000.

> *Total costs for the treatment of disease, medical errors, drug reactions, and hospital-caused infections is 1 trillion dollars annually!*
>
> ———♛———

The total direct costs for the treatment of disease and the direct costs related to medical errors, drug reactions, and hospital-caused infections is 1 trillion dollars annually!

Medicine is a big money machine; don't let anyone tell you otherwise. Modern medicine is filled with political posturing, power grabbing and high rollers. Just consider: *The pharmaceutical industry makes money off of sickness and disease* and certainly does not want publicity from drug-related deaths. Modern medicine is primarily chemical-based health care. Even though it helps many people, it also harms and kills hundreds of thousands of people every year. The statistics cannot be denied.

The Gary Null study released in July 2004 estimated that nearly 800,000 people die from a combination of drug reactions, medical mistakes, unnecessary surgeries and infections developed after being treated in a hospital. If that many die, two to three times that many are harmed but are fortunate enough to survive. It is staggering to realize that the very system put into place to heal us is actually causing the deaths of thousands upon thousands of people each year.

I vividly remember first reading about the Top Ten Killers and coming to a shocking and exhilarating conclusion. *My patients were almost never suffering or dying from these diseases.* I was shaken! For twenty years I had been practicing as a chiropractor, helping my patients deal with back and neck pain, easing their headaches and giving them lifestyle advice to improve their health. But chiropractic care was much more than those things: it was having monumental effects on quality of life and longevity.

The irony was not lost on me. Chiropractors – as well as other natural health care providers – have been called quacks, unscientific cultists and medical charlatans for decades by the American Medical Association, yet *their* methods are unintentionally killing people in unprecedented numbers.

As excited as I was to realize that my patients were experiencing exceptional health, this revelation was immediately followed by a heart-wrenching conclusion: Most people were clearly dying from preventable diseases.

With further reading and research I became thoroughly convinced that most people who succumb to one of the Top Ten Killers die well before their God-appointed time. Have you ever been to the funeral of a loved one who died of cancer or a heart attack and heard someone say, "I guess it was just his/her time"? No way! People are not supposed to die from cancer, strokes and heart attacks or any of the other Top Ten Killers. It simply is not God's will for us to suffer these horrible, painful deaths.

Most people who succumb to one of the Top Ten Killers die well before their God-appointed time.

Each of the Top Ten Killers is an absolutely horrible way to die. Almost all of them are drawn out and filled with suffering. The good news is that they are preventable![32] You do not have to dread dying the way most Americans do, from heart disease, cancer, stroke or any of the other Top Ten. As you follow the wisdom and advice outlined in this book, you can look forward to a lifetime of divine health filled with purpose and joy followed by a peaceful transition into eternity when your God-ordained days are fulfilled.

> *ord, it is sobering to see how people are dying needlessly from sickness and disease when this was never a part of your plan. Fill me with compassion for those who are suffering and the resolve to pursue a different path – one of divine health and healing. Thank you that I do not have to dread the Top Ten Killers, but that with your guidance and strength I can make wise choices to keep those diseases from claiming my life. I praise you and bless your name. Amen.*

---

32   With the possible exception of unintentional injuries, which are largely beyond our control.

The Top Ten Killers
– In Review

- THE TOP TEN KILLERS CLAIM THE LIVES OF 8 OUT OF EVERY 10 PEOPLE PREMATURELY. THEY ARE:

    1. HEART DISEASE

    2. CANCER

    3. STROKE

    4. LUNG DISEASES

    5. UNINTENTIONAL INJURY

    6. DIABETES

    7. ALZHEIMER'S

    8. FLU AND PNEUMONIA

    9. KIDNEY DISEASE

    10. SEPTICEMIA/SEVERE INFECTIONS

- ADVERSE DRUG REACTIONS ACTUALLY DESERVE THE TITLE OF THE NUMBER ONE KILLER IN THE UNITED STATES.

- DEATH DUE TO DOCTORS AND MEDICAL PROCEDURES DESERVES A PLACE ON THE TOP TEN KILLER LIST AS WELL.

- ALMOST EVERY SINGLE TOP TEN KILLER IS PREVENTABLE.

- IT IS NOT GOD'S WILL FOR HIS PEOPLE TO DIE FROM ANY OF THE TOP TEN KILLERS.

Think of the funerals you have attended lately. How many of those loved ones died as a result of one of the Top Ten Killers? _____

_____

_____

After you learned of someone's death to cancer or another of the Top Ten Killers, have you ever heard a loved one say, "It was just their time"? What is your reaction to this theory? __

_____

_____

_____

_____

_____

Do you know anyone who died at an old age due to "natural causes?" _____

_____

Do you know anyone personally who has had an adverse reaction to a prescription medication? _____

_____

_____

_____

Do you know anyone personally who has died as a result of a doctor's error? _____

_____

_____

_____

Notes: _____

_____

_____

_____

_____

_____

_____

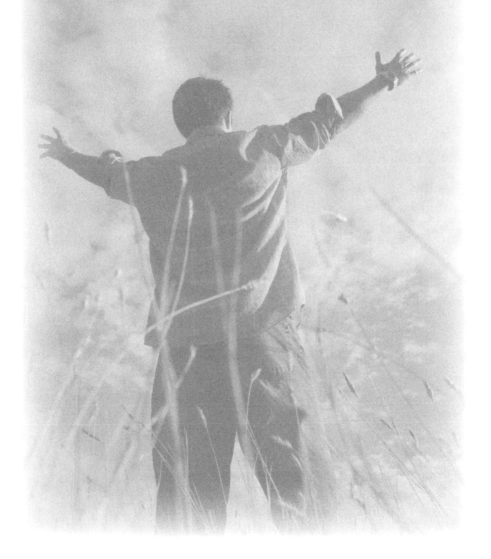

God heals, and the doctor takes the fee.

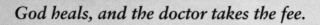

BENJAMIN FRANKLIN

Chapter Fourteen

A Sorry State of Affairs

W E LIVE IN THE GREATEST nation in the world and quite possibly in all of history. I hope that your heart swells as mine does every time you hear the national anthem being sung at a baseball game or you watch the American flag being raised above our Olympic athletes. We are truly blessed to be living at this time in history in this wonderful country.

I wish I could boast so freely about the state of health care in our nation, but the unfortunate truth is that the health of our citizens is not just mediocre – it is downright pitiful. We live in a society where health disorders and disease are the norm — where many preventable and unnecessary deaths occur every single day. The majority of our citizens consume prescribed drugs on a daily basis to treat chronic disease and/or pain. The state of our society's health is at an all-time low.

> *The majority of our citizens consume prescribed drugs on a daily basis.*
>
> ——ᴡ——

The reason for this is simple and tragic: the healthcare system in our nation is not a healthcare system at all. It is a "sick care" system. The medical community is designed to treat illness rather than prevent it and even these efforts are at best mediocre.

The financial toll on our country is staggering. According to the World Health Organization, Americans spend an average of $7026 per person per year for health care. This amounts to over two trillion dollars – almost 20 percent of the nation's gross domestic product. The cost of health care in our nation exceeds that of any other country in the world.

You would think the high price tag would result in improved health, but sadly, that is not the case. We have a higher infant mortality rate than most other developed nations. We rank 34th in life expectancy and 29th in infant mortality, tied with Slovakia and Poland.[33] And according to the Center for Disease Control, 7 out of 10 deaths are the result of a chronic disease.

Consider these sobering medical statistics:

ᴡ ACCORDING TO THE AMERICAN HEART ASSOCIATION, HEART DISEASE IS AN UNDERLYING CONTRIBUTING CAUSE IN 58 PERCENT OF ALL ADULT DEATHS. 910,000 PEOPLE WILL DIE THIS YEAR FROM CARDIOVASCULAR DISEASE – ONE LIFE WILL BE CUT SHORT EVERY 35 SECONDS.

---

33   Dyman, Jackson. "The Sorry State of American Health." <u>Time Magazine.</u> December 1, 2008: 41-51.

TREATMENT OF HEART DISEASE WILL COST $403.1 BILLION.

❦ TREATMENT OF DIABETES COSTS OUR NATION 132 BILLION DOLLARS EVERY YEAR.[34]

❦ ACCORDING TO THE AMERICAN STROKE ASSOCIATION, A STROKE OCCURS EVERY 45 SECONDS AND KILLS 157,000 PEOPLE PER YEAR. 700,000 AMERICANS WILL SUFFER A NEW OR RECURRENT STROKE THIS YEAR, AND 5.5 MILLION OF OUR CITIZENS HAVE ALREADY EXPERIENCED ONE. STROKE TREATMENT COSTS $57.9 BILLION ANNUALLY.

❦ ACCORDING TO THE AMERICAN CANCER ASSOCIATION, 564,700 AMERICANS DIE FROM CANCER EVERY YEAR, MAKING IT THE SECOND LEADING CAUSE OF DEATH IN OUR NATION. THE LIFETIME RISK OF DEVELOPING CANCER IS 1 IN 2 FOR MEN AND 1 IN 3 FOR WOMEN. CANCER TREATMENT COSTS $74 BILLION ANNUALLY.

❦ INTERESTINGLY ENOUGH, THE STARBUCKS CORPORATION SPENDS MORE ANNUALLY ON HEALTH COSTS THEN THEY DO FOR COFFEE BEANS!

Sickness care and emphasis on treatment instead of wellness care is bankrupting us as a nation. We are a great country with more access to doctors, hospitals, fancy medical procedures and prescription drugs than any other nation on the planet. Why aren't we healthy? *Because we are reacting to disease instead of preventing it. And because, quite frankly, this approach is a huge mistake.*

> *Sickness care and emphasis on treatment instead of wellness care is bankrupting us.*

---

34   American Heart Association

Mistakes in health care? You bet! Barbara Starfield, M.D. of the John Hopkins School of Hygiene and Public Health recently published an article in The Journal of the American Medical Association. She stated that doctors' errors are the third leading cause of death, making them responsible for at least 250,000 deaths annually including 12,000 from unnecessary surgeries, 7000 due to medication errors in hospitals, 20,000 from other errors in hospitals, 80,000 due to hospital acquired infections and 106,000 from the non-error, negative effects of prescription drugs.

The total direct costs for the treatment of disease and the direct costs related to medical errors, drug reactions and hospital-caused infections is 1 trillion dollars. These figures are just the financial facts. They do not even begin to capture the millions of people who actually suffer from disorders and disease or the grieving family members who watch a loved one struggle to survive.

The system is broken and I am afraid it will not be fixed anytime soon. That leaves the responsibility up to us as individuals to educate ourselves and makes decisions that will keep us "Fit for the King." Believers who walk in divine health and healing can steer clear of the broken healthcare system that is trying so hard and failing miserably in so many ways. God has provided a better way and it is available to you and me!

L ord, thank you that I do not have to rely on anyone else to walk in wholeness and I can be free of disease, sickness and pain. Thank you for giving me every good thing that I need to walk in divine health and healing. I pray that you would open my eyes to the changes that need to be made in my life and habits so that I can joyfully live every day you have ordained for me. I bless you and praise your name! Amen.

A Sorry State of Affairs
– In Review

- ⚜ WE LIVE IN A GREAT NATION – WITH MEDIOCRE LEVELS OF HEALTH.

- ⚜ THE AMERICAN HEALTHCARE SYSTEM IN OUR NATION IS NOT A HEALTHCARE SYSTEM AT ALL. IT IS A "SICK CARE" SYSTEM. THE MEDICAL COMMUNITY IS DESIGNED TO TREAT ILLNESS RATHER THAN PREVENT IT.

- ⚜ THE FINANCIAL COSTS OF TREATING SICKNESS ARE STAGGERING.

- ⚜ THE COST TO PEOPLE'S LIVES IS EVEN MORE SOBERING.

- ⚜ MISTAKES MADE BY HEALTHCARE PROVIDERS ARE THE THIRD LEADING CAUSE OF DEATH. DOCTORS ARE RESPONSIBLE FOR AT LEAST 250,000 DEATHS ANNUALLY DUE TO ERRORS.

- ⚜ THE HEALTHCARE SYSTEM IS BROKEN AND WILL NOT BE FIXED ANYTIME SOON. IT IS EVERY INDIVIDUAL'S RESPONSIBILITY TO DO EVERYTHING IN THEIR POWER TO MAINTAIN AND PROTECT THEIR OWN HEALTH AND PROMOTE DIVINE HEALING.

Which would you say is more common: to hear someone boast about their good health or complain about their poor health?

_____

_____

Are you surprised at the health of Americans? Do you expect our nation to be healthier because we are a leader in the world?_____

_____

_____

Does spending more money on healthcare than any other nation in the world suggest that we should also be healthier than any other nation? _____

_____

_____

Do you sense that our healthcare system is focused on reacting to diseases and disorders instead of preventing them?_____

_____

_____

Have you ever experienced a medical error?_____

_____

_____

Have you ever had a loved one suffer or even die as a result of a medical error?_____

_____

_____

Has this chapter convinced you that your health is your responsibility and should not be delegated to anyone else? ____

_____

_____

_____

_____

_____

Notes: _____

_____

_____

_____

_____

_____

_____

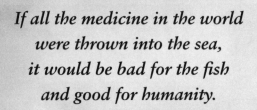

*If all the medicine in the world
were thrown into the sea,
it would be bad for the fish
and good for humanity.*

Oliver Wendell Holmes, M.D.

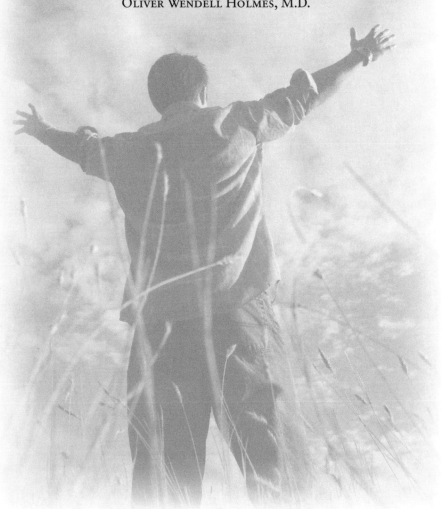

Chapter Fifteen

Debunking the Drug Myth

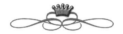

A S A NATURAL HEALTH CARE PROVIDER I have a love/hate relationship with the medical profession and the pharmaceutical industry. On one hand, I am grateful for life-saving emergency medicines and medical care. There are glorious moments when skilled and passionate doctors and nurses step in and save the lives of their patients. I am thankful for these dedicated men and women. On the other hand, I am horribly frustrated by the medical and pharmaceutical industries' attempts to fix everything with pills, pills and more pills. Instead of focusing on prevention and wellness, we live in a society that believes that taking drugs makes us healthier. But does taking drugs make a person healthier?

Our society is dominated by an archaic mindset — a method of thinking that teaches us from a very early age to reach for a chemical solution to all of life's ills, ailments and pains; whether they are physical or emotional. This thinking

> *Nearly 80 percent of people over the age of 45 are regularly using prescription drugs.*
> ꝏ

has created a whole nation addicted to caffeine, tobacco, alcohol, illegal drugs and prescription drugs – a society with drive-thru drug windows that has been taught to reach for a chemical every time they need or want to feel better. Medication usage is epidemic. According to an AARP study, nearly 80 percent of people over the age of 45 are regularly and currently using prescription drugs.[35]

Every single day this mindset leaves a swath of destruction and devastation that far exceeds all natural disasters combined. Deaths attributed directly to prescription drugs events alone range somewhere between 299-1000 people per day depending on whose statistics you believe. The impact includes lives lost, suffering caused and financial costs far greater than all tsunamis, earthquakes and tornadoes combined.

This pervading mentality promotes treatment of symptoms versus correction of cause and gives no credence to prevention whatsoever. Even when the medical profession attempts to address disease prevention the answer is a drug or vaccine. Preventive medicine at best is early detection of a disease that is already present. It is absolutely shameful that Prevention magazine (which is dedicated to disease prevention and healthcare) is filled with more drug ads than health articles!

---

35   Prescription Med Usage, AARP March 2002

The medical establishment erroneously concludes that the introduction of chemicals into the human body cures all or nearly all disease and improves health. Drugs are great when absolutely necessary, but they are not the solution to our nation's monstrous health problems. For chronic health problems, drugs simply do not work. Though they may temporarily alleviate pain, lower blood pressure or artificially bring cholesterol levels down, they do not fix the underlying problem causing the symptoms.

Every week we have the wonderful privilege of consulting with patients who come to our practice. Many of them seek us out in desperation because they are struggling with health problems that no one has been able to diagnose or treat effectively. Most of these patients are

> *It is nearly impossible to tell which symptoms are real and which are side effects.*

literally taking handfuls of pills — so many pills, in fact, that it is nearly impossible to tell which symptoms are real (from their health issue) and which are side effects of the medications.

The typical patient over age 50 that comes into our practice is taking four to five different prescription medications, and it is not uncommon to see others who take many more. I recently began treating a nurse who was actually taking 16 different medicines daily, multiple times per day. The patient who holds the record in my practice for the most medication was taking *29 different prescription medicines!* The sad news is that despite all of the drugs, these patients are still very sick people.

Nearly thirty years of private practice and personally caring for 20,000 patients has led me to the firm conclusion that *drugs do not correct health problems.* When they do appear to be working, drugs are only chemically stimulating or inhibiting functions in the body. For example, if a person develops high blood pressure they are routinely prescribed medication to treat it. If drugs actually fixed the high blood pressure, they should only need to be taken for a specific period of time, the problem would be solved and the patient would be free to discontinue the meds. In truth, as soon as a person stops taking their high blood pressure medicine their blood pressure goes right back up, because *medication does not get to the root of the problem.* It only chemically covers it up.

Medication does not get to the root of the problem.

The same scenario is true for nearly every kind of drug on the market, which is why patients are on so much medication for an indefinite period of time. Their problems are never fixed and they continually need more and more drugs to cover up the symptoms of deteriorating health. There is never an end in sight. "Once prescribed, forever needed" is the rule rather than the exception.

Then there are the side effects. Look at the side effects list of one common cholesterol-lowering statin drug. Keep in mind that (1) billions of dollars are spent on this type of cholesterol-lowering drug every year, including the doctors' visits and blood tests required by their use, (2) that there is very little evidence in drug trials on people without heart disease that statin drugs reduce deaths or serious health events,[36] and (3) there are many natural, effective methods of lowering cholesterol without drugs. This is a list of the more serious side effects listed in the fine print of a popularly-prescribed statin drug:

PANCREATITIS	ANXIETY
HEPATITIS	DEPRESSION
JAUNDICE	NERVOUSNESS
LIVER DAMAGE	PSYCHIC DISTURBANCES
LIVER FAILURE	MEMORY LOSS
CIRRHOSIS	TREMORS
LIVER CANCER	LOSS OF SEX DRIVE
INSOMNIA	IMPOTENCE

Who wants to sign up for that? Some of you unknowingly already have!

Adding to the questionability of prescription drugs are some of the methods of the pharmaceutical industry itself. Drug companies highly compensate the very researchers who do the efficacy studies on their products. This practice is widespread in both the pharmaceutical industry and the medical profession and the FDA tolerates it. In the case of statin drugs, Dr. Rodney Hayward, Professor of Internal Medicine at the University of Michigan Medical School, says, "It's almost impossible to find

---

36   Carey, John. "Do Cholesterol Drugs Do Any Good?" Businessweek January 28, 2008. Pages 52-59.

Drug companies make medications appear much more effective than they really are.

☗

someone who believes strongly in [cholesterol-lowering] statins who does not get a lot of money from the [drug] industry."[37]

Drug companies also make their medications appear much more effective than they really are. A recent ad by Pfizer proclaims that "Lipitor (a statin drug) reduces the risk of heart attack by 36 percent*.... in patients with multiple risk factors for disease."

Do not overlook any asterisks or fine print in a drug advertisement! If you look more closely at the research cited in fine print, you will discover that 100 people took the drug for 3 1/3 years and a control group of 100 people took a sugar pill for the same amount of time. Of the 100 people taking the sugar pill, three had hearts attacks. Of the 100 people taking the actual drug, two had heart attacks. The resulting 36 percent statistic sounds impressive, but the truth is that to spare just one person a heart attack, 100 people had to take a drug with substantial potential side effects for 3 1/3 years. The remaining 99 folks in the study got no measurable benefit.[38]

This calculation is know as the NNT for a drug, or the "number needed to treat" for one person to benefit. This little-known statistic is quite useful in determining a drug's actual effectiveness.

---

37   Ibid.

38   Carey, John. "Do Cholesterol Drugs Do Any Good?" <u>Businessweek</u> January 28, 2008. Pages 52-59.

If 200 people have to take a drug to see a benefit for just one person, is the drug actually worth the risk? Statin drugs often have an NNT of 250 or more *for low risk patients!* [39]

Dr. Jerome R. Hoffman, Professor of Clinical Medicine at the University of California at Los Angeles, poses just that question. "What if you put 250 people in a room and told them they would each pay $1,000 a year for a drug they would have to take every day, that many would get diarrhea and muscle pain, and that 249 would have no benefit? And that they could do just as well by exercising?" It takes no stretch of the imagination to determine how people would respond to that scenario if they knew the facts up front.

Drug companies continually exaggerate their claims, understate side effects and highly compensate their researchers and spokespersons. The FDA is aware of the questionable practices of pharmaceutical companies as they highly compensate their researchers and spokespeople.

> *Drug companies highly compensate their researchers and spokespersons.*

Drugs, politics and money can indeed be a toxic combination. Drugs are big business. Unfortunately, they are not solving the health crisis that Americans are finding themselves in; in fact, drugs are actually compounding people's health problems. Dr. Ray Strand, M.D., states, "The use of prescription medication is the third leading cause of death in the U.S."[40]

---

39   Ibid.

40   Strand, Ray D., M.D., (2003). Death by Prescription. Nashville, TN: Thomas Nelson, Inc.

We used to think of the Food and Drug Administration (FDA) as a friend and protector but that view is severely in question. According to Dr. Strand,

> *Half of all the side effects are discovered after the drug is released for public use.*

fewer than 56 percent of all side effects from a new drug are discovered during a drug's clinical trials. That means that *half of all the side effects are discovered after the drug is released for public use.* You are the clinical trial for a new drug! Dr. Strand recommends that you avoid taking any drug that has not been on the market at least five years. It is no wonder so many new "wonder drugs" become debacles and are taken off the market when people start dying or having severe side effects.

If you are still not convinced that drugs are big business, consider this: Glaxo Smith Kline and its co-maker Bayer signed a *$20 million deal* with the National Football League to promote their drug Levitra to compete with Viagra (the leading erectile dysfunction drug). Pfizer sponsors a car on the NASCAR circuit. CBS's Morley Safer was reportedly paid six figures for one day in the studio to make videos that resembled newscasts but were really drug promotional spots to be shown during local TV newscasts. Astra Zeneca spent a half billion dollars to convince consumers to switch from Prilosec to Nexium ("the purple pill"). All of this according to Marcia Angell, M.D., in her book *The Truth About Drug Companies*.[41] She is the former editor-in-chief of the New England Journal of Medicine and is currently a member of Harvard Medical School's Department of Social Medicine. Dr. Angell goes on to write:

> The pharmaceutical industry has an iron grip on Congress and the White House. It has the largest lobby in Washington – with more lobbyists than there are elected representatives in Congress – and contributes heavily to political campaigns.
>
> Drug companies promote disease to match their drugs. Millions of normal Americans have come to believe that they have dubious or exaggerated ailments like "generalized anxiety disorder," "erectile dysfunction," "PMDD," and "GERD."
>
> Drug companies have enormous influence over what doctors are taught about drugs and what they prescribe.
>
> Drug companies have substantial control over clinical trials of their drugs. There is good reason to believe that much of the company-supported research on prescription drugs is biased as a result.[42]

Equally troubling are the hundreds of thousands of patients who experience adverse drug events (ADEs). ADEs may be the result of allergic reactions, severe side effects and reactions with other medications. USA Today reported in 2005 that the number of adverse drug events reported to the U.S. Food

---

41   Angell, Marcia, M.D., (2004). The Truth About Drug Companies: New York, NY, Random House.

42   Ibid.

> *Drugs should always be a last resort when every natural and less invasive method has been attempted.*
>
> ———❦———

and Drug Administration reached an all-time high in 2004. There were almost half a million ADE reports made by pharmaceutical companies, health professionals and patients, a 14 percent increase over reports in 2003.

While the FDA requires drug manufacturers to file ADE reports, health professional's reports are voluntary, leading government officials to believe that the reported number represents only a portion of the actual ADEs experienced by patients.

People cannot be drugged into better health. Drugs should always be a "fourth down and punt" solution – a last resort when every natural and less invasive method has been attempted and life-saving measures must be taken.

Take a few moments and consider your own attitude toward medication:

- ❦ HOW QUICK ARE YOU TO TAKE A PILL WHEN YOU EXPERIENCE PAIN OR ILL HEALTH? ARE YOU WILLING TO WAIT A WHILE TO SEE IF IT PASSES ON ITS OWN?

- ❦ HOW BIG IS YOUR PERSONAL STOCKPILE OF PRESCRIPTION AND OVER-THE-COUNTER MEDICATION?

- ❦ WHEN YOUR CHILDREN GET SICK HOW QUICKLY TO YOU GIVE THEM MEDICATION OR CALL THE DOCTOR? DO YOU PRAY FOR THEIR HEALING FIRST? (CONSIDER HOW YOUR REACTION INFLUENCES THEIR ATTITUDE TOWARD MEDICATION.)

Here are some guidelines for lowering the risk of drug reactions and interactions:

1. *Always ask your doctor if there are any more natural alternatives you can try before using a drug.*

2. *Inform all of your doctors of all prescription and over-the-counter drugs and herbal products you are taking.*

3. *Carry a complete and current list with you at all times in case of an emergency. The list should include the name of each drug or herbal product, recommended dosage and frequency, date started and doctor who prescribed it.*

4. *Ask your doctor and pharmacist questions. Show them your current drug and herb list. Ask if any of the medications you are taking are contraindicated (meaning that they should not be taken together).*

5. *Always ask for an explanation of the most common side effects.*

6. *Ask how soon you should expect to see results.*

7. *If the drug(s) do not seem to be working after a few days or you develop any new symptoms, call your doctor and ask if you should continue to take the medication.*

8. *Read the information insert in the package. If there is none, ask the pharmacist for a printout of the drug's actions, interactions, side effects and contraindications.*

9. *Take medications exactly as directed.*

10. *Most importantly, make significant lifestyle changes that will allow you to eliminate the root of the problem and eventually stop the drug(s) altogether. These might include*

losing weight, starting a disciplined eating and exercising program and consulting a chiropractor, nutritionist or other alternative healthcare provider.

Living on medication is not what Jesus had in mind when he said, "I have come that you might have life and have it more abundantly."[43] The abundant life is waking up every day pain-free, full of energy, completely rested and charged up to go out and do what you do for Jesus! You have better options than spending the rest of your life taking handfuls of pills every day.

> *Living on medication was never what Jesus had in mind.*

---

43   John 10:10

Lord, thank you that you are the Truth and that you delight to reveal truth to your children. I pray that you would continue to give me wisdom and discernment as I make decisions that will lead to divine health and the healing of my health issues. Convict me of ways that I have been depending on medication and doctors instead of depending on you. Heal me. Give me wisdom, guidance and direction to understand the root of my heath problems. Empower me to pursue treatments that come from your hand instead of just from a pill bottle. Thank you for providing methods of treatment that will solve my health problems and bring health and healing to my body. I praise your name! Amen.

Debunking the Drug Myth
– In Review

- ☙ EMERGENCY MEDICINES AND MEDICAL CARE ARE A BLESSING.

- ☙ THE MEDICAL PROFESSION'S ANSWER TO TREAT HEALTH ISSUES IS ALWAYS DRUGS.

- ☙ DRUGS MAY TEMPORARILY TREAT THE SYMPTOMS, BUT THEY DO NOT GET TO THE ROOT CAUSE OF HEALTH ISSUES.

- ☙ PEOPLE WHO TAKE DRUGS CONTINUE TO SUFFER FROM DETERIORATING HEALTH, EVEN IF THE DRUG IS MASKING THEIR PROBLEM.

- ☙ DRUGS ARE ACCOMPANIED BY A LONG LIST OF POTENTIAL AND DANGEROUS SIDE EFFECTS.

- ☙ DRUG COMPANIES HAVE VERY QUESTIONABLE PRACTICES, INCLUDING PAYING RESEARCHERS AND SPOKESPERSONS.

- ☙ DRUG COMPANIES COMMONLY EXAGGERATE RESEARCH IN THEIR CLAIMS OF A DRUG'S EFFECTIVENESS.

- ☙ BECAUSE HALF OF ALL THE SIDE EFFECTS ARE DISCOVERED AFTER THE DRUG IS RELEASED FOR PUBLIC USE, YOU ARE THE CLINICAL TRIAL FOR A NEW DRUG!

- ☙ HUNDREDS OF THOUSANDS OF PATIENTS EXPERIENCE ADVERSE DRUG REACTIONS (ADEs) EVERY YEAR.

- ☙ PEOPLE CANNOT BE DRUGGED INTO BETTER HEALTH. DRUGS SHOULD ALWAYS BE A "FOURTH DOWN AND PUNT" SOLUTION – A LAST RESORT WHEN EVERY NATURAL AND LESS INVASIVE METHOD HAS BEEN ATTEMPTED AND LIFE-SAVING MEASURES MUST BE TAKEN.

- ☙ IF YOU MUST TAKE DRUGS, THERE ARE MANY THINGS YOU CAN DO TO LOWER THE RISK OF DRUG REACTIONS AND INTERACTIONS.

- ☙ DRUGS ARE NOT SOLVING THE AMERICAN HEALTH CRISES, DESPITE THE FACT THAT THEY ARE BEING PRESCRIBED IN EVER-INCREASING NUMBERS.

How many prescription drugs are you currently taking each day? List them here. Are all of your doctors aware of all the medications you are taking? _____

_____

_____

Have those medications completely solved your health issues or are they simply treating the symptoms? (Can you expect to ever stop taking them because the problem has been solved?)

_____

_____

_____

Are you experiencing any side effects from your medications? List them here._____

_____

_____

Are you experiencing any unexplained symptoms that might be side effects of the medication you are currently taking?___

_____

_____

_____

Stop for a moment and read the fine print on your prescriptions. Do they include an NNT number? (Number needed to treat.) Ask your pharmacist for this information for each prescription drug you are taking._____

_____

_____

_____

Make an appointment to see a wellness practitioner. Ask for treatment options that are natural and work out a plan to gradually move from medicine-based healthcare to natural healthcare. _____

_____

_____

_____

Notes: _____

_____

_____

_____

_____

_____

_____

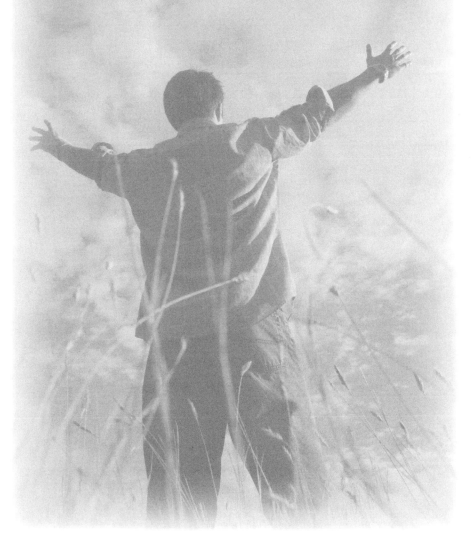

*Unhappiness is not knowing
what we want and killing ourselves to get it.*

DON HEROLD

Chapter Sixteen

Ruling and Reigning Over Stress

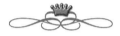

MANY EXPERTS BELIEVE that 90 percent of all health problems are directly or indirectly linked to stress. Consider these statistics:

American Stress Statistics

- 54% of Americans are concerned about their levels of stress.

- 73% name money as their #1 stress factor.

- More than 50% suffer adverse health effects from stress.

- Stress is linked to the six leading causes of death.

- 23% of women executives and professionals feel "super-stressed."

- 19% of male executives and professionals feel "super-stressed."

- ♛ 54% say stress causes them to fight with others.
- ♛ 40% report their job is "very" or "extremely" stressful.
- ♛ 30% say they are "often or "always" under stress at work.
- ♛ 25% have felt like screaming or shouting due to stress.
- ♛ 14% felt like striking a co-worker in the past year.
- ♛ 12% have called in sick because of job stress.
- ♛ $300 billion spent annually on stress-related medical expenses, absenteeism and health insurance costs.

Source: The American Institute of Stress, American Psychological Association

Truthfully, we will never be totally free from stress until we go to be with Jesus, and some of the stress that we experience in life is good and even necessary. Consider how the stress of providing for our families motivates us to get up for work on mornings we would rather sleep in. Newborns add a new level of stress to our lives as well, but we recognize the blessing of our children. Our bodies are actually wonderfully designed to tolerate quite a bit of stress, and that is good news. The answer to stress is not trying to rid our lives of it but to handle it effectively with God's help.

> *We will never be totally free from stress until we go to be with Jesus.*
> ♛

I generally see two groups of patients in my practice. The first group pursues health and wellness proactively, bringing their whole family in for spinal adjustments and wellness advice, all of which promote long-term, life-long health. The second group of patients usually sees me *after* they have started experiencing tension, pain or disease in their body. These folks are generally tense and fatigued and are most often exhibiting physical, mental and emotional symptoms due to the stress in their lives.

Speaking personally, I am not immune to stress any more than you are. I perform a juggling act each day, balancing the responsibilities of being a Christian, husband, lover, father, son, uncle, mentor, leader, author, consultant, doctor, speaker, employer, taxpayer, educator, businessman and friend. Each one of us has unique and multiple roles to play in life, all of which are very important. The challenge we face is how to manage it all and keep our health and our sanity intact? The answer is a concept called "margin."

Margin is the space that exists between us and our limits. It is the gap between rest and exhaustion, between health and sickness. Having margin means leaving the house in the morning and arriving at the office on time despite hitting every red light on the way. Margin supplies us with the space, time and resources to arrive fresh, relaxed and ready for life even when things do not go quite as we planned.

In his book *Margin*, Richard A. Swenson, M.D., describes our problem as "margin-less living." He addresses the peril of over-stretching, over-loading and over-booking our lives. Instead, we are encouraged to "....break our addiction to getting ahead and being better off."

The idea of slowing down, doing less and increasing margin in our lives is extremely countercultural. Every day we are pushed and prodded into being more, doing more and earning more. In fact, it has been said that if the devil cannot make you be bad, he will just make you busy!

I will admit it: I have to constantly keep myself from always wanting to do "just one more thing" before leaving for work in the morning. I start the day with good intentions but too often use up my "get to work early" margin accomplishing just one more task before walking out the door. This forces me to race through yellow lights, exceed the speed limit and burst into the office rushing to make it on time. On the glorious days when I honor the margin I have built into my schedule, I arrive relaxed, energized and fresh, eager to serve my staff and my patients. What a difference that extra time makes!

In our struggle to get everything done, when is enough, enough? I recently met a stressed-out single parent who has her seven-year-old enrolled in ice skating lessons, a basketball league, dance classes and swimming lessons, all at the same time. I understand her good intentions in wanting her daughter to learn valuable social and life skills but fear that she does not realize the added stress and strain all these activities heap upon their family. We had a rule when our children were young that neither of our children was allowed to be involved in more than two extracurricular activities at any one time. This helped to keep margin (and sanity) in our after-school and weekend schedules. I would encourage you to adopt a similar guideline in your home as well.

In the same way, when is enough money enough? In the struggle to get ahead financially, build the retirement account or fill the college savings coffer, we too often push ourselves closer and closer to the breaking point. If there is no margin in our finances it increases the urgency to accomplish more, work harder, make more sales, get to one more appointment or make one more phone call before ending a long, stressful day on the job.

We spend the first third of our lives educating ourselves so that we can go out and earn a good living. We spend the middle third of our lives working hard to earn the good living and saving for

> *When is enough money enough?*

our children's college education and our retirement, hoping to enjoy the final third of our lives in comfort and relaxation. Too often, though, we arrive at retirement after years of stress and physical neglect in such bad shape physically that our golden years are spent treating various maladies and diseases instead of enjoying that wonderful stage of life.

In the early years we spend our health getting money for retirement, and then we spend our retirement funds trying to get our health back. Stress is a vicious cycle that will not change without determination and wise choices. The results of stress and pushing to the limits are sobering and the payoff is staggering. Years of cramming in more and more stress into our lives results in failed health, broken marriages and disintegrating family relationships.

> *Too often our golden years are spent treating maladies and diseases instead of enjoying that wonderful stage of life.*
>
> ❦

There is good news! Great health is equal to great wealth, and we really do not have to compromise our health in order to achieve financial wealth. We may have to work smarter, re-evaluate our goals or the timeframes in which we achieve those goals, but *there is a better way to live.*

Your health is your single greatest asset. Without it, nothing else matters very much. Do not let stress destroy the plans God has for you to live a long, prosperous life.

Lord, thank you for revealing areas in my life that are robbing me of good health. I confess that many times I cram my schedule full without regard for margin. I give your Holy Spirit permission to point out activities that are adding to my stress and diminishing the time I need to rest and relax. Please help me to establish my priorities in a way that is pleasing to you, brings glory to your name and sanity to my life. Thank you that stress will no longer rule and reign over me but that I will walk in divine health every day of my life. Amen.

Ruling and Reigning Over Stress
– In Review

- ♛ MANY EXPERTS BELIEVE THAT 90 PERCENT OF ALL HEALTH PROBLEMS ARE DIRECTLY OR INDIRECTLY LINKED TO STRESS.

- ♛ STRESS IS A VICIOUS CYCLE THAT WILL NOT CHANGE WITHOUT DETERMINATION AND WISE CHOICES.

- ♛ THE ANSWER TO STRESS IS NOT TRYING TO RID OUR LIVES OF IT BUT TO HANDLE IT EFFECTIVELY WITH GOD'S HELP.

- ♛ MARGIN IS THE SPACE THAT EXISTS BETWEEN US AND OUR LIMITS. IT IS THE GAP BETWEEN REST AND EXHAUSTION, BETWEEN HEALTH AND SICKNESS.

- ♛ THE IDEA OF SLOWING DOWN, DOING LESS AND INCREASING MARGIN IN OUR LIVES IS EXTREMELY COUNTERCULTURAL.

- ♛ YOUR HEALTH IS YOUR SINGLE GREATEST ASSET. WITHOUT IT, NOTHING ELSE MATTERS VERY MUCH.

- ♛ DECREASING THE LEVEL OF STRESS IN YOUR LIFE IS A STEP IN THE DIRECTION OF DIVINE HEALTH AND HEALING.

Can you relate to any of the American Stress Statistics listed at the beginning of this chapter? List a few of your top stressors here. _____

_____

_____

_____

_____

_____

Which sounds simpler to you: To reduce stress *before* it becomes problematic in your life or to treat the effects of stress *after* your health is negatively impacted?_____

_____

_____

If you had to grade yourself on how well you are dealing with stress levels in your life, what grade would you get? Have you created margin in your daily schedule? _____

_____

_____

_____

_____

Do you have enough margin in your finances? How can you create more margin to lower your financial stress? _____

_____

_____

_____

_____

How much margin have you created in your health? What is the first thing you should do to create more? _____

_____

_____

_____

Notes: _____

_____

_____

_____

_____

_____

_____

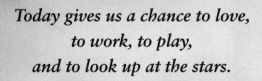

Today gives us a chance to love,
to work, to play,
and to look up at the stars.

HENRY VANDYKE

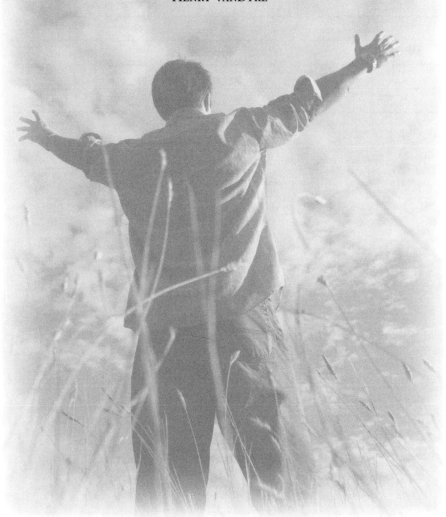

Chapter Seventeen

Establishing Priorities

CHOOSING TO REDUCE and manage the stress in your life is an extremely important choice that requires a good deal of self-discipline. Setting aside some time to step back and get an objective view of the "big picture" of your life can give you great insight into lowering stress and re-ordering your priorities.

I have found a great illustration that I enjoy sharing in my seminar and "Fit for the King" church wellness programs.[44] I take a large one-gallon glass jar and tell the audience that the jar represents their life, with a limited amount of space for all of their activities. I fill it two-thirds full with white rice, which represents life's less important obligations and distractions, including things like watching TV, mowing the lawn, pulling the weeds, driving the kids to school, doing the laundry, etc. Then

---

44   For more information on the "Fit for the King" church wellness program, visit www. SettingThingsStraight.com.

I pour small marble-sized rocks into the jar until it is about 75 percent full. The rocks represent more important obligations such as time spent at work earning a living, at school getting educated, going to church on Sundays and eating breakfast, lunch and dinner, all of which are important.

Lastly, I hold up four tennis balls, each one representing a very important priority necessary to living a contented, meaningful Christian life.

> **God** – For Christians, God is not a priority, He is *The Priority*. I do not want to get to the end of my life and stand before God regretful of the way I spent my time. My ultimate goal in life is to hear Him say, "Well done, good and faithful servant."[45] To maintain a vibrant relationship with the King of my life, I need to spend time reading the word, praying, meditating and conversing with Him every day. Jesus always took time to spend connecting with His Father, and so should we.[46]

> **People** – This includes the most precious people in your life (your family) as well as others that are important to you (friends, neighbors, clients, coworkers, etc.). Jesus always took time for people no matter how busy He was. People and relationships take time but pay us back with incredible joy and are the source of great meaning in our lives.

> **Joy** – There is an important difference between joy and happiness. Happiness is dependent on my circumstances

---

45 Matthew 25:21

46 "Very early in the morning, while it was still dark, Jesus got up, left the house and went off to a solitary place, where he prayed." Mark 1:35

at any given moment. I am happy when my checking account balance is high, when I drive a new car off the dealer's lot and when my wife and kids are healthy. Joy, however, is the result of the hope I have in Jesus and my faith in Him. It is based on the complete assurance that God is in control and that He loves me like crazy regardless of how I feel, the bills I might owe, how stressed I am or how many pounds I need to lose. Joy is based on the hope I have in Him. As a follower of Christ, I know that whatever may befall me in this life, I am destined for eternal life with God in heaven. What a wonderful truth to cling to in the midst of our constantly changing circumstances! Happiness is nice, but my constant prayer is for joy to fill my heart every moment of the day.

Mission and Purpose — I believe that every single person has a God-given calling, something special that God has uniquely hard- and soft-wired them to do. He has custom designed you with the perfect combination of strengths, skills, talents and abilities to accomplish those things that only you can do on the earth while you are here. I do not know about you, but I want my life to count. I want to know that the thousands of hours I spent getting my degree mattered in somebody's life. Most of all, I want to accomplish everything I can in this life for Jesus, my King. *I want to live long and strong for Him.*

As I hold up each tennis ball and talk about the four priorities, the audience quickly realizes my dilemma: there simply is not enough room for the balls in the jar. The most important priorities have been pushed aside in favor of distractions and obligations.

Just when everyone thinks the illustration is finished, I grab a second one-gallon glass jar of equal size. This time I put the four tennis balls in *first*. Then I add an equal amount of rocks and shake the jar. On top of that goes the same amount of white rice (representing the dishwashers that need to be emptied, the snowy driveways that need to be shoveled, the walls that need another coat of paint and all the distractions of life), which all settles to the bottom with extra room to spare. The conclusion? When we make time for what is most important in our lives and trust God to do the rest, there is always room (margin) left over for all the "fun stuff" that life offers. In Matthew 6:33 Jesus said it this way: "But seek first his kingdom and his righteousness, and all these things will be given to you as well." You can trust Him to do just that!

> *Strive to live each day as if it were your last.*

In his book *When the Game Is Over, It All Goes Back in the Box,* author John Ortberg refers to this stunning visual illustration, stating, "The jar only comes in size 24. It cannot be super-sized." God created our day with 24 hours and gives us the opportunity to spend it as we will.

Strive to live each day as if it were your last. Schedule your days, weeks, months and years according to what is really important. The average life expectancy is 28,740 days. The problem with averages is that some of us will live longer, but many of us will die sooner. At the end of your life will you regret how you spent your time or look back with pride and satisfaction? It is your choice.

Take a hard look at the following four critical areas of your life and bring them back into balance. Ask yourself the following questions:

w HEALTH HABITS

- Are you feeding your body constructive superfoods?

- Do you get regular exercise?

- Are you eliminating troublesome habits that are robbing you of good health?

- Are you maintaining good spinal health with regular chiropractic adjustments?

- Are you getting adequate rest each night?

w SPENDING HABITS

- Are you frequently stressed due to finances?

- How much margin have you built into your monthly finances?

- Where could you cut back on spending to lower your stress?

- Are you giving generously to the Lord?

- When was the last time you took a close look at your personal budget?

- Where are you spending money needlessly or wastefully?

- Could you downsize your mortgage or car payment(s) to build more margin into your finances?

♛ Spiritual Habits

- Are you too busy to pray? (If so, you are too busy!)

- Are you putting God first according to Matthew 6:33?[47]

- Have you overcommitted yourself with spiritual responsibilities?

- When was the last time you prayed with your spouse?

- What extracurricular activities could you cut out or reorganize to allow more time for daily devotions?

♛ Relationship Habits

- Have you considered that your relationship with God is your most important relationship?

- Is there anyone with whom you need/want to spend more time with but cannot seem to find the time?

- Who do you need to spend less time with due to their negative influence on your attitude/outlook?

- When was the last time you and your spouse took a romantic weekend getaway?

- When was the last time you had a date night with your spouse?

By making more intentional decisions about these critical areas and building margin into each one, you will free up more time for other pursuits and will drastically lower your stress level at the same time.

---

47   "But seek first his kingdom and his righteousness, and all these things will be given to you as well." Matthew 6:33

We are too busy not to pray, to play, or to stay "Fit for the King." There is a lot at stake. How well will a pastor be able to shepherd his flock if he is stricken with high cholesterol, high blood pressure and ultimately a heart attack or stroke? How well can we parent or grandparent if we are ill or under the influence of prescription drugs each and every day? We cannot perform at our best when we push ourselves to the limit at every turn. If you wear out your body, where are you going to live?

> *We are too busy not to pray, to play, or to stay "Fit for the King."*

God does not want you to be stressed. He wants you to care about what is important and submit your worries and fears to Him.[48] Do not allow stress to rob you of the peace and good health God has planned for your life.

Making the hard choice to focus only on the important "stuff" and letting the other things take care of themselves will greatly improve the quality of your existence and allow an inner peace and freedom to pervade your life. It will also help you to stay healthy and to stick around so that you can accomplish all the tasks the Lord has for you. It will help you to live out every day God has ordained for you to live. Do not allow the devil to steal even one hour from your life!

---

48   "….casting all your care upon Him, for He cares for you." 1 Peter 5:7

Thank you, Lord, that I do not have to live my life full of worry and stress. Help me to set my priorities according to your will and your Word, trusting you with the outcome. Give me the self discipline to keep my priorities in order and restore margin to each area of my life. Make my work productive and my rest enjoyable, and may each bring glory to your Name. Show me creative ways to build margin back into my life. Amen.

Establishing Priorities
– In Review

- ☙ CHOOSING TO REDUCE AND MANAGE THE STRESS IN YOUR LIFE IS AN EXTREMELY IMPORTANT CHOICE THAT REQUIRES A GOOD DEAL OF SELF-DISCIPLINE.

- ☙ THERE ARE FOUR VERY IMPORTANT PRIORITIES NECESSARY TO LIVING A CONTENTED, MEANINGFUL CHRISTIAN LIFE:
  1. GOD
  2. PEOPLE
  3. JOY
  4. MISSION AND PURPOSE

- ☙ THESE FOUR PRIORITIES MUST BE SCHEDULED *first* IN ORDER TO GIVE THEM THE PRIORITY THEY DESERVE AND TO KEEP THEM FROM BEING CROWDED OUT BY LESS IMPORTANT TASKS.

- ☙ CHRISTIANS SHOULD ESTABLISH THEIR PRIORITIES SO THAT AT THE END OF THEIR LIFE THEY WILL LOOK BACK WITH PRIDE AND SATISFACTION AND FEEL NO REGRET.

- ☙ THERE ARE FOUR CRITICAL AREAS OF A CHRISTIAN'S LIFE THAT NEED TO BE BALANCED:
  1. HEALTH HABITS
  2. SPENDING HABITS
  3. SPIRITUAL HABITS
  4. RELATIONSHIP HABITS

- ☙ BY MAKING MORE INTENTIONAL DECISIONS ABOUT THESE CRITICAL AREAS AND BUILDING MARGIN INTO EACH ONE, TIME IS FREED UP FOR OTHER PURSUITS AND STRESS LEVELS ARE DRASTICALLY REDUCED AT THE SAME TIME.

- ☙ GOD DOES NOT WANT HIS PEOPLE TO BE STRESSED.

One a scale of 1 to 10, how stressful would you say your life is? _____

_____

Do you find yourself so busy taking care of the small things in life (errands, chores, etc.) that you end up neglecting the big things (relationships, God, your God-given calling)?_____

_____

_____

_____

_____

Do you sense that stress is having a negative impact on your health? _____

_____

_____

Do you have margin in your finances? In your health? In your spiritual life? In your relationships? Or are you so busy that there is no extra time, energy or resources to dedicate to those areas? _____

_____

_____

_____

Review this chapter, choosing a few practical ways to reduce the stress in your life. Put those ideas into practice this week.

_____

_____

_____

_____

Notes: _____

_____

_____

_____

_____

_____

_____

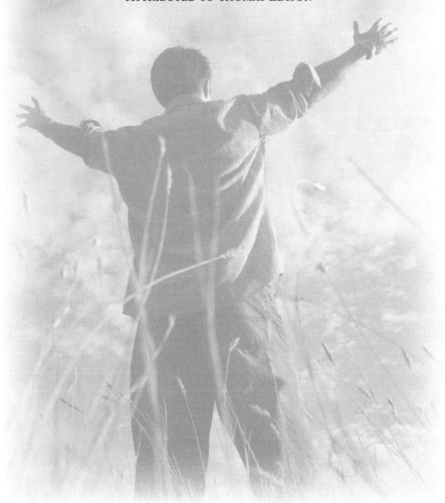

The doctor of the future will give no medicine
but will interest his patients in the care
of the human frame, in diet and in the
cause and prevention of disease.

ATTRIBUTED TO THOMAS EDISON

Chapter Eighteen

The Best-Kept Health Secret

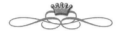

WE HAVE DETERMINED THAT GOD wants you to walk in divine health and that physical, emotional and spiritual health will allow you to fulfill His pre-ordained plan for your life. We have also discussed how your body's innate or inborn ability to heal itself is a large part of divine health. In this chapter, I want to share with you what I believe is *the best-kept health secret and single most overlooked aspect of healing.*

Your body is organized into ten different systems:

System	Function
Nervous	Controls and communicates with every system, tissue, organ and cell in the body.
Cardiovascular	Food and oxygen transport. Includes the heart, veins, arteries and capillaries.
Respiratory	Brings air into the body, providing oxygen for each cell and disposing of carbon dioxide.
Digestive	Breaks down food into useable nutrition for cells, organs and tissues.
Reproductive	Produces the ability to conceive and bear children.
Endocrine	System of glands which produce hormones and enzymes to stimulate and control various body functions.
Skeletal	Composed of bones, ligaments and tendons. It works with the muscular system to move the body. Provides support and protection for organs.
Muscular	Tendons and muscles that work in conjunction with the skeletal system to move the body.
Excretory	Eliminates waste from the body.
Immune	Protects the body. Fights off infection and disease. The defense system of the body.

While all of these systems are important and necessary for proper function of the body, the nervous system is in control of them all and coordinates all of their functions. The nervous system is composed of three parts:

1. Brain –

The brain is the supercomputer that controls every single function in the body. It generates and sends millions of nerve messages down your spinal cord every day.

<u>Subconscious control</u> – Most of the nerve impulses sent by the brain are done subconsciously. You breathe, your eyes blink and your heart beats without any conscious thought. Almost all of your internal functions are controlled subconsciously by your autonomic (automatic) nervous system.

Your heart beats on average 72 times a minute. Every second or so, a nerve impulse is sent from the heart regulation center in the brain down the spinal cord to the heart, signaling it to beat once more. If you stood up and ran around the house, your brain would recognize a higher need for oxygen and added nutrition and would tell your heart to pump faster, sending oxygenated blood to your muscles to meet the demand. All of this control is performed without your conscious thought.

<u>Conscious Control</u> – Other brain signals are sent because you make conscious demands on your body. For example, you can blink your eyes quickly by just thinking about it. Your body moves on command by consciously deciding to move in a certain direction.

Your brain is responsible for *every* function in your body, including your body's ability to heal itself. *Great healing starts in the brain!*

2. *Spinal Cord*

The spinal cord is hidden in a tunnel on the inside of your spine. It is about as big around as your index finger and extends from the base of your skull all the way down to your waistline. This "super-highway" carries millions of nerve impulses from your brain to every cell in your body. The impulses travel at 270 miles per hour!

Your spine is made up of 24 spinal bones, or vertebrae. The vertebrae fit together like puzzle pieces stacked one on top of another, providing support for your upper body and acting like a protective tunnel around the spinal cord. The spine was designed to be flexible, allowing you to bend, twist and turn.

3. *Nerves*

Between each vertebra are small openings that serve as doorways for nerves to exit the spine. These nerves carry electrical messages from the brain, down the spinal cord and out to each part of the body. Nerves are the roads or network that nerve impulses travel on to reach their destination. If you were to open up your body and take a look, you would see that the nerves in your body resemble flesh-colored spaghetti noodles. The largest nerve is the sciatic nerve. It is actually ribbon-like, about as wide as your little finger and runs from the lower back down the back of the knees to your feet, branching off into smaller nerve pathways along the way. As nerves travel farther away from the spine they get smaller and smaller until they are actually microscopic once they reach the surface of the skin. But no matter how tiny they get, every single cell in your entire body is connected to your brain through these nerve pathways.

The following table lists just some of the functions of each nerve:

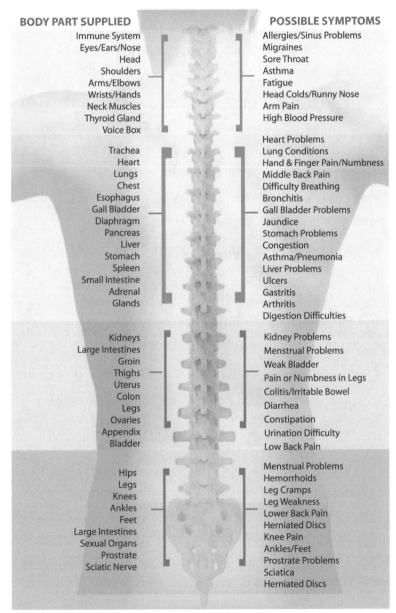

BODY PART SUPPLIED	POSSIBLE SYMPTOMS
Immune System	Allergies/Sinus Problems
Eyes/Ears/Nose	Migraines
Head	Sore Throat
Shoulders	Asthma
Arms/Elbows	Fatigue
Wrists/Hands	Head Colds/Runny Nose
Neck Muscles	Arm Pain
Thyroid Gland	High Blood Pressure
Voice Box	
	Heart Problems
Trachea	Lung Conditions
Heart	Hand & Finger Pain/Numbness
Lungs	Middle Back Pain
Chest	Difficulty Breathing
Esophagus	Bronchitis
Gall Bladder	Gall Bladder Problems
Diaphragm	Jaundice
Pancreas	Stomach Problems
Liver	Congestion
Stomach	Asthma/Pneumonia
Spleen	Liver Problems
Small Intestine	Ulcers
Adrenal	Gastritis
Glands	Arthritis
	Digestion Difficulties
Kidneys	Kidney Problems
Large Intestines	Menstrual Problems
Groin	Weak Bladder
Thighs	Pain or Numbness in Legs
Uterus	Colitis/Irritable Bowel
Colon	Diarrhea
Legs	Constipation
Ovaries	Urination Difficulty
Appendix	Low Back Pain
Bladder	
	Menstrual Problems
Hips	Hemorrhoids
Legs	Leg Cramps
Knees	Leg Weakness
Ankles	Lower Back Pain
Feet	Herniated Discs
Large Intestines	Knee Pain
Sexual Organs	Ankles/Feet
Prostrate	Prostrate Problems
Sciatic Nerve	Sciatica
	Herniated Discs

SPINAL NERVE CHART

If you were to take out all of your nerves and lay them end to end, they would extend nearly 12 miles! Something to think about the next time you hear someone say, "You've got nerve!" It is these nerves and the messages traveling over them that control all of your body's functions and its amazing ability to heal itself.

You can see why proper, optimal function of the spine and nervous system is necessary for the health and function of every other system in the body. Nothing happens in your entire body apart from your nervous system. The best-kept secret of divine health is maintaining a properly-aligned, fully-functioning spine and nervous system.

Maintaining proper alignment in your spine is the best way to insure the perfect flow of nerve impulses between your brain and your body. Now that you know the secret of nervous system health, the next chapter will reveal how to keep your nervous system functioning as God intended it to.

Lord, thank you once again for how wonderfully you created my body. Thank you for each system and the amazing way they work together. Thank you for revealing the importance of the spine and nervous system health and for giving me the opportunity to pursue the divine health that you intended for me. You are a giver of good gifts, and I accept good health and healing from your hand! Empower me by your Holy Spirit to make the choices and changes that will lead me into better and better health. Amen.

The Best-Kept Health Secret – In Review

❧ YOUR BODY IS ORGANIZED INTO TEN DIFFERENT SYSTEMS:

1. NERVOUS

2. CARDIOVASCULAR

3. RESPIRATORY

4. DIGESTIVE

5. REPRODUCTIVE

6. ENDOCRINE

7. SKELETAL

8. MUSCULAR

9. EXCRETORY

10. IMMUNE

❧ OF ALL THESE SYSTEMS, THE NERVOUS SYSTEM IS THE MOST IMPORTANT BECAUSE IT CONTROLS AND COORDINATES ALL THE OTHERS.

❧ THE NERVOUS SYSTEM IS COMPOSED OF THREE PARTS:

1. BRAIN – THE SUPERCOMPUTER THAT CONTROLS EVERY FUNCTION OF THE BODY.

2. SPINAL CORD – THIS "SUPER-HIGHWAY" CARRIES MILLIONS OF NERVE IMPULSES FROM THE BRAIN.

3. NERVES – CARRY ELECTRICAL NERVE MESSAGES FROM THE BRAIN OUT TO EVERY CELL IN THE BODY.

- ♛ PROPER, OPTIMAL FUNCTION OF THE SPINE AND NERVOUS SYSTEM IS NECESSARY FOR THE HEALTH AND FUNCTION OF EVERY OTHER SYSTEM IN THE BODY.

- ♛ THE BEST-KEPT SECRET OF DIVINE HEALTH IS MAINTAINING A PROPERLY-ALIGNED, FULLY-FUNCTIONING SPINE AND NERVOUS SYSTEM.

Review the list of the ten systems in your body. Are you experiencing health problems in any of these systems? _____

_____

_____

_____

Have you considered that the improved function of your nervous system will improve your health in every other system?

_____

_____

_____

_____

When was the last time you had your spine and posture examined for proper alignment? _____

_____

_____

Are you committed to the pursuit of nervous system health in order to improve your total quality of health? _____

_____

_____

Notes: _____

_____

_____

_____

_____

_____

_____

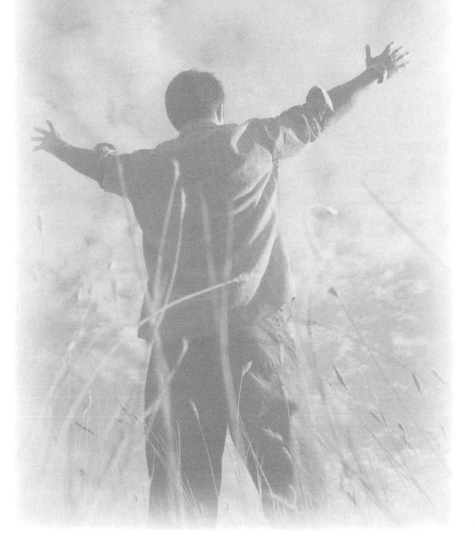

Oh the nerves, the nerves;
the mysteries of this machine called man!

———◆———

CHARLES DICKENS

Chapter Nineteen

You've Got Nerve

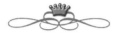

NOW THAT WE KNOW THE BASICS about the parts of the nervous system, let us take a look at how communication between the brain and the body actually works.

Between each vertebra is a tiny opening about the size of the end of a pencil called the "vertebral foramen." ("Foramen" is Latin for "hole.") A nerve impulse generated by the brain comes shooting down the spinal cord and exits out one of the spinal nerves, which carries it to its destination. How nerve impulses know which spinal level to exit is still a mystery. Nerve signals going to different regions of the body know exactly which spinal nerve exit to take to arrive at the correct destination within milliseconds of leaving the brain. The impulse travels to its destination and relays the message from the brain and initiates proper function. These nerve messages are the foundation for health, healing and function for every part of the body.

The spinal column is made up of 24 individual spinal bones (or vertebrae). It is a wonderful feat of engineering on the part of our Creator. The spinal bones are able to move and shift, allowing us to bend, turn and twist our bodies. Unfortunately, the verterbrae are susceptible to misalignment. When a spinal bone shifts out of its normal position, we call it a *subluxation,* which means "minor dislocation." When a vertebra shifts out of normal alignment, the nerve opening (foramen) becomes smaller, crowding and squeezing the nerve as it passes through. Over time the nerve becomes irritated and the proper flow of nerve impulses is blocked. Instead of 100 percent nerve flow, the electrical nerve signals become weakened. This interruption in nerve flow is called "nerve interference."

The spinal column is made up of 24 individual spinal bones.

Subluxations (misalignments of the spinal bones) can occur for any number of reasons, including:

- Lifting improperly.

- Childbirth – Think of how a baby's head is twisted and wrenched as they are delivered. Delivery can also subluxate a mother's spine and pelvis.

- Sports injuries and impacts. (This is how I was introduced to chiropractic.)

- Unhealthy sleeping positions, including using a pillow that is too thick or too thin, sleeping on your stomach or even falling asleep in the armchair watching late night TV.

- ♛ Jarring car accidents – The average person experiences one car accident every 10 years.

- ♛ Slips and falls.

- ♛ Repeated falling as toddlers learn to walk.

- ♛ Poor posture.

- ♛ Repetitive activities such as assembly line work, sitting at a computer for prolonged periods of time, etc.

- ♛ Stress – As neck, shoulder and back muscles tighten under stress, they pull on the vertebra, pulling them out of proper alignment.

- ♛ Chemical stress on the body from a poor diet, food additives and medications can also cause subluxations.

Stress is the number one cause of subluxations in the spine. Stop and consider where you usually feel stress in your body. We typically feel tension and pain in our neck and shoulders, our back, tension in the scalp and headaches. Because of the dense muscular attachments to the bones of the spine, the vertebrae (spinal bones) can get pulled out of alignment rather easily from the muscular effects of stress.

> *The spine is the switchboard of the nerve system.*

More seriously, since the spine is the switchboard of the nerve system, alignment problems in the spine open the door to impacting our inner health as well. The nerves, which run through and exit out between the bones of the spine, literally control the functions of our entire body. Whether the misalignment resulted from the muscular effects of stress, a car accident, lifting injury, strain from the birth process, or a slip or fall, subluxations cause a serious threat to our health on a daily basis. Though regular spinal care through chiropractic does not eliminate the stress, chiropractic care effectively minimizes the effects that stress has on our bodies and keeps us healthier.

Imagine that one summer evening you go into the backyard to water the garden. You drag the hose to your tomato plants and turn it on but just a trickle of water comes dripping out. Walking around the side of the house you quickly discover the culprit: you have inadvertently parked the car on the hose. A quick parking job restores the free flow of water and your tomato plants can now receive all the water they need to remain happy and healthy.

The squashed garden hose is a good illustration of how a subluxation affects the nerves exiting the spine. If a subluxated vertebra is interfering with the nerve messages telling your heart to beat, imagine the result on your heart health. How well do you think your heart will continue working over time? In the same way, how well can your brain control your blood pressure or the flow of blood through the arteries and veins of your heart if it is unable to communicate with the heart due to the nerve interference caused by subluxations? This is often how heart problems and heart disease first start.

Every organ and system in your body can be affected by subluxation.

Every organ and system in your body can be affected by subluxation and the resulting nerve interference in this way. If your pancreas receives limited nerve messages it may result in diabetes.[49] Subluxations in the top two vertebrae at the base of the skull frequently result in allergies, sinus problems, asthma and other breathing problems. Arthritis, back problems, numbness and headaches are other very common symptoms of subluxation.

The problem is simple to understand but very few people are aware it even exists. Subluxations in your spine are very serious, and the greatest danger is that you usually cannot feel them. This is largely because *only 10 percent of subluxations cause pain.* Ninety percent of the population walks around suffering from all types of sickness and maladies without ever considering that their health problems are the result of misalignment in their spines. For those ten percent who experience spinal pain from subluxations, the pain is actually a blessing because it alerts you to the problem of spinal misalignment.

Only 10 percent of subluxations cause pain.

If you go to a medical doctor because of heartburn, he or she is likely to prescribe a little purple pill. This drug is designed to stop heartburn and indigestion by decreasing the amount of acid produced by your stomach. The heartburn may go away

---

49   There is very little research to support this statement; however, chiropractors observe this clinically on a regular basis. Diabetic patients often see improvement of their condition after chiropractic care is begun.

but this "solution" just stops the symptoms without correcting the true cause of the problem. Your stomach was designed to produce stomach acid in order to digest your food. You may be heartburn-free but are now faced with a new problem: decreased digestion and the resulting nutritional deficiencies that result from poorly digested food.

Now let us assume you go to a chiropractor for the same heartburn. The first thing he or she would do is check your spine in the area that supplies nerve messages to your stomach to make sure it is properly aligned. These nerves exit the spine between your shoulder blades. If misalignment is found affecting the nerves that control digestion, there is now an explanation for the symptoms you are experiencing. Once the spinal bones are put back into place, nerve messages to your stomach will flow more freely, correcting the root of the problem and eventually ending the heartburn. This corrects the source of the problem without subjecting your body to all of the side effects that come with prescription medication. Subluxations block healing in the body. Spinal adjustments release healing. The body is best able to heal itself when the nerve connections are open and there is unhindered flow of nerve messages.

A healthy, well-aligned spine allows the full uninhibited flow of brain messages to each part of your body.

A healthy, well-aligned spine allows the full uninhibited flow of brain messages to each part of your body. Throwing prescription drugs at the problem is like unplugging the warning light on the dashboard of your car and pretending there is not a problem — or pulling the battery out of a screeching smoke alarm and ignoring the fire as it rages through your home. It might make the annoying symptoms go away, but it does not correct the source of the problem.

When your spine is properly aligned and the nervous system is able to work at full capacity there are two wonderful results:

1. *There is correct function of each organ and system as the brain is able to control and regulate them properly.*

2. *The body's ability to heal itself and maintain ongoing good health is enhanced.*

The following list is a summary of the benefits of long-term chiropractic care. These have been documented by multiple research studies and are routinely observed by chiropractors and their patients worldwide.

People who receive regular chiropractic care:

- HAVE HIGHER RESISTANCE TO DISEASE/STRONGER IMMUNITY

- GET FEWER CHILDHOOD DISEASES (I.E. CHICKEN POX, MEASLES AND MUMPS)

- TAKE FEWER PRESCRIPTION DRUGS

- REPORT IMPROVED QUALITY OF LIFE

- HAVE FEWER HOSPITAL AND NURSING HOME ADMISSIONS

- HAVE 50 PERCENT REDUCTION IN MEDICAL DOCTOR VISITS

- REDUCE MEDICAL COSTS ON AVERAGE BY TWO THIRDS

- REPORT BETTER SLEEP, IMPROVED LOVE LIFE

- ♛ SENIORS HAVE BETTER MOBILITY AND GREATER WALKING STABILITY

- ♛ NOTICE IMPROVED MENTAL AND EMOTIONAL HEALTH

- ♛ ENJOY GREATER LIFE SATISFACTION AND CONTENTMENT

- ♛ EXPERIENCE IMPROVED ATHLETIC PERFORMANCE

- ♛ EXHIBIT LOWER STRESS LEVELS AND REDUCED TENSION

- ♛ GET SICK LESS OFTEN AND RECOVER FASTER

- ♛ EXPERIENCE LESS TIME LOST FROM WORK

- ♛ HAVE AN IMPROVED SENSE OF WELL-BEING

- ♛ FEEL STRONGER, WALK BETTER, TRAVEL EASIER

- ♛ EXPERIENCE GREATER OVERALL HEALTH

I have personally seen chiropractic care release what almost seems like supernatural healing ability in thousands of my patients. I have seen kidney function return, carpal tunnel syndrome eliminated and diabetes and thyroid issues resolved. A handful of my patients have lost 40 to 50 pounds without any change in their diet or lifestyle simply because their thyroid was at last able to function properly. Many of my male patients no longer experience high blood pressure or erectile dysfunction, and female patients have seen a balancing of their hormones that has eased symptoms of menopause, hot flashes, PMS and painful, heavy periods. People's level of health nearly always improves on any number of levels once they begin chiropractic care. When the spine and body are lined up properly as God designed them to be, our bodies are able to return to normal function the way He originally intended.

Regular chiropractic care is one of the most effective methods of preventing and avoiding the Top Ten Killers[50]. As we learned previously, disease occurs in places of weakness. Organs and tissues that are deprived of the free flow of nerve impulses are functioning in a weakened state. Chiropractic care enables the body to function the way God designed it to – in vibrant health and with the fullest potential for healing. People who see a chiropractor and get their spines checked and realigned on a consistent basis clinically have much lower incidences of heart attacks, strokes, cancer and other illnesses.[51] Much research is needed to understand the connection between a healthy spine, improved health and lessened disease, but the clinical improvements and observations that chiropractors see occur in their offices every day are undeniable.

> *Regular chiropractic care is one of the most effective methods of preventing and avoiding the Top Ten Killers.*

If you are not currently seeing a chiropractor or have never had your spine checked, I urge you to do so as soon as possible. New research continually points out the benefits of spinal care, and you will never experience complete health and healing in your body apart from a fully functioning spine and nervous system. Your body will thank you with more vibrant divine health and renewed healing ability.

---

50   This statement has not been evaluated by the FDA.

51   Ibid.

Father, thank you for the wonderful design of my nervous system. Thank you that you created me to walk in divine health and innate healing. Please help me to take advantage of every opportunity to promote health in my body, mind and spirit. May every cell, tissue and organ in my body work at full function to bring glory to your name each day, and let my vibrant health and joyful spirit be a testimony to your goodness. Amen.

You've Got Nerve
– In Review

- ❦ NERVE IMPULSES GENERATED BY THE BRAIN COME SHOOTING DOWN THE SPINAL CORD AND EXIT OUT THE SPINAL NERVES, WHICH CARRIES IT TO ITS DESTINATION.

- ❦ WHEN A VERTEBRA SHIFTS OUT OF NORMAL ALIGNMENT, THE NERVE OPENING (FORAMEN) BECOMES SMALLER, CROWDING AND SQUEEZING THE NERVE AS IT PASSES THROUGH. THIS IS CALLED "SUBLUXATION."

- ❦ NINETY PERCENT OF SUBLUXATIONS DO NOT CAUSE ANY PAIN, WHICH MEANS THAT MANY GO UNNOTICED AND UNCORRECTED.

- ❦ SUBLUXATIONS CAN OCCUR FOR ANY NUMBER OF REASONS, BUT THE RESULT IS INHIBITED NERVE FLOW ("NERVE INTERFERENCE") TO THE BODY.

- ❦ EVERY ORGAN AND SYSTEM IN YOUR BODY CAN BE AFFECTED BY SUBLUXATION AND THE RESULTING NERVE INTERFERENCE. OVER TIME, LIMITED NERVE FLOW RESULTS IN LIMITED FUNCTION OF THE DESTINATION CELLS AND ORGANS.

- ❦ DOCTORS TREAT THE RESULTING SICKNESS, PAIN OR DISEASE WITH PRESCRIPTION MEDICATION, WHICH MAY EASE THE SYMPTOMS BUT DOES NOT ADDRESS THE ROOT OF THE PROBLEM. THE PRESCRIPTION DRUGS USED TO TREAT THE PROBLEM COME WITH KNOWN AND UNKNOWN SIDE EFFECTS WHICH WILL AFFECT THE PATIENT'S HEALTH IN MANY OTHER WAYS.

- ♛ CHIROPRACTIC CARE CORRECTS THE ROOT OF THE PROBLEM NATURALLY, WHICH DECREASES SYMPTOMS AND RESTORES HEALTH.

- ♛ THE BODY IS BEST ABLE TO HEAL ITSELF WHEN THE NERVE CONNECTIONS ARE OPEN AND THERE IS UNHINDERED FLOW OF NERVE MESSAGES.

- ♛ WHEN YOUR SPINE IS PROPERLY ALIGNED AND THE NERVOUS SYSTEM IS ABLE TO WORK AT FULL CAPACITY THERE ARE TWO WONDERFUL RESULTS:

    1. THERE IS CORRECT FUNCTION OF EACH ORGAN AND SYSTEM AS THE BRAIN IS ABLE TO CONTROL AND REGULATE THEM PROPERLY.

    2. THE BODY'S ABILITY TO HEAL ITSELF AND MAINTAIN ONGOING GOOD HEALTH IS ENHANCED.

- ♛ MULTIPLE RESEARCH STUDIES HAVE DOCUMENTED THE BENEFITS OF ROUTINE CHIROPRACTIC CARE.

- ♛ CHIROPRACTIC CARE ENABLES THE BODY TO FUNCTION THE WAY GOD DESIGNED IT TO – IN VIBRANT HEALTH AND WITH THE FULLEST POTENTIAL FOR HEALING.

Browse through the list of possible causes of subluxations. Are there any that you have personally experienced? _____

_____

_____

_____

Consider the prescription medications you may be taking. Do you sense that they may be treating your symptoms while ignoring the root cause of your medical problem? _____

_____

_____

_____

What side effects are you experiencing from prescription medications that may be compromising your health in other areas? ___

_____

_____

_____

Have you ever seen a chiropractor? What was your experience?

_____

_____

_____

_____

What friends or family members see a chiropractor and would be willing to share their experience with you? Start looking for a highly qualified doctor of chiropractic today. _____

_____

_____

_____

Notes: _____

_____

_____

_____

_____

_____

_____

_____

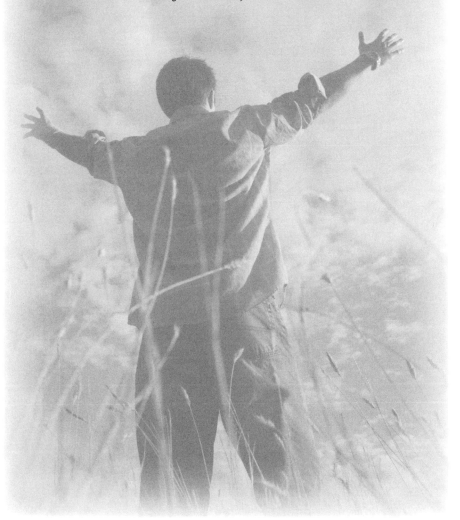

*Sickness is looked upon by most people
as inevitable. If we live for health and seek health
instead of disease, we find it.*

—◈◈◈—

J.H. Tilden, M.D.

Chapter Twenty

Becoming a Healthier You

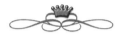

MODERN MEDICINE'S UNDERSTANDING of sickness is based on the Germ Theory of Disease. The germ theory states that sickness and disease are the result of coming in contact with a germ, such as a bacteria or a virus. Medicine has always taken an outside-in approach to health, blaming outside factors for causing disease. If the germ theory were true, no one who works in a hospital would be alive to talk about it; all the doctors and nurses would die as a result of daily contact with germs. After all, they work in the most germ-ridden environment that exists on the planet. The hospital is where the sickest of the sick are taken.

> *If the germ theory were true, no one who works in a hospital would be alive to talk about it.*

We all know doctors and nurses who are enjoying good health. Why do they stay healthy despite breathing in all those germs? Why do *we* stay healthy despite touching bacteria-laden door knobs, showing affection to one another and sharing tight quarters on bus and train commutes?

Let us look at three myths about health and sickness and the facts behind them:

MYTH #1   WHEN YOU FEEL GOOD YOU ARE HEALTHY.

Fact: Your health is not based on how you feel. People who feel good drop over dead every day from heart attacks, aneurysms and strokes.

MYTH #2   GERMS, BACTERIA AND VIRUSES FLOAT AROUND;
YOU "CATCH" THEM AND GET SICK.

Fact: Germs only cause sickness when a person's immune resistance is decreased. Just as Jerusalem had strong, thick walls to keep out invaders, your immune system constantly fights germ invaders. It is only when the strength of your immune system is compromised that you succumb to germs and get sick. Subluxations in the spine are one of the biggest causes of lowered immunity. In addition, a poor diet, lack of exercise, lack of sleep and high stress levels also lower your immunity and make you susceptible to sickness.

MYTH #3   DRUGS, SURGERY AND DOCTORS MAKE YOU WELL.

Fact: Drugs, surgery and doctors assist in healing, but only your body can heal itself according to God's divine design.

A Brief History of Chiropractic Care

On September 18, 1895, Dr. Daniel David Palmer performed the first recorded chiropractic adjustment on Harvey Lillard, a janitor who worked in the same building as Dr. Palmer in Davenport, Iowa. Mr. Lillard, who had complained of hearing problems for over seventeen years, allowed Dr. Palmer to examine his spine. At the time, Dr. Palmer had been studying the cause and effect of disease. He had discovered a lump on Mr. Lillard's back and suspected a vertebra was out of place. He repositioned the vertebra with a gentle thrust. After several such treatments, Mr. Lillard's hearing was completely restored.

Since this first chiropractic adjustment, the art and science of chiropractic has progressed, with advanced diagnostic procedures, sophisticated equipment and scientific research.

A spinal adjustment is the procedure a chiropractor uses to correct your spine and remove subluxations. Getting your spine adjusted is a simple, comfortable procedure that only takes a few minutes each visit. The doctor examines the patient through x-ray, posture analysis, palpation (examining by touching with one's hands) and often thermal imaging. After reviewing the test results with the patient, a treatment plan is then determined which generally includes multiple and repeated spinal adjustments over a course of months to correct the misalignments in the spine. (Think of chiropractic care as "orthodontics" for the spine.)

The patient normally lies down, fully dressed in their street clothes on a special padded table known as an "adjusting table" that allows them to rest and breathe comfortably. The doctor locates the vertebrae that are out of alignment and uses his or her hands or an adjusting instrument to gently press the vertebrae back into better alignment. Sometimes the bones make a quiet noise as they move into proper position but this differs with each patient. Regardless, chiropractic adjustments should never be painful or uncomfortable.

Chiropractic care is the largest natural healing profession on the planet.

Chiropractic care is one of the fastest growing methods of health care and is the largest natural healing profession on the planet. Everyone can benefit from spinal adjustments to either regain their health or to maintain it. Chiropractic care is a life-long approach to health and well being. A healthy spine means a healthier you.

A secondary benefit of chiropractic care that is just starting to garner attention is how it can lower the cost of health care in general.

When Chiropractors Act as Primary Care Providers, Costs Drop

A study in the May 2007 issue of the Journal of Manipulative and Physiological Therapeutics reports health plans that use Chiropractors as Primary Care Providers (PCPs) reduce their health care utilization costs significantly.

The study covered the seven-year period from 1999 to 2005. Researchers compared costs and utilization data from an Independent Physicians Association (IPA) that uses Chiropractors as PCPs [primary care physicians] and a traditional HMO [Health Maintenance Organization] that doesn't.

The Chiropractic PCPs had 59 percent fewer hospitalizations, 62 percent fewer outpatient surgical cases and 85 percent lower drug costs compared with the HMO plans.

The patients in the Chiropractic PCP group also reported higher satisfaction with their care than the HMO group. Over the seven-year period, Chiropractic patients consistently demonstrated a high degree of satisfaction with their care that ranged from 89 percent to 100 percent.

Study co-author James Winterstein, D.C. says that patients using Chiropractic PCP health care groups "experienced fewer hospitalizations, underwent fewer surgeries and used considerably fewer pharmaceuticals than HMO patients who received traditional medical care."

> *The Chiropractic PCPs had 59 percent fewer hospitalizations.*

"The escalation of medical expenditures remains an urgent problem in the United States and it's becoming quite clear that cost containment strategies by conventional medical providers are failing to achieve even mediocre results," he said. "This study confirms that the integration of [medical], chiropractic and other complementary and alternative medicine (CAM) providers can positively impact patient quality of care while limiting costs. This approach to patient care has great potential to improve the U.S. healthcare system."

I strongly urge you to seek a qualified, passionate chiropractor and start investing in your health with regular spinal adjustments. Here are some ideas to help you find the best chiropractor in your area.

How to Find an Excellent Chiropractor

You would not pick a surgeon out of the yellow pages to remove your appendix, nor should you haphazardly choose a chiropractor. Every profession consists of men and women with varying levels of passion and expertise, and chiropractors are no different. When you search for a chiropractor, the goal is to find the best in your area.

There are many good referral sources including pastors, dentists, personal trainers and the staff of health food stores in your area. Ask them for the name of the best chiropractor in town. If you know people who already see a chiropractor, ask about their experience. Would they "highly" recommend their chiropractor to you? Ask what they specifically like about him or her.

Once you have a few good recommendations, call the chiropractic offices and ask these questions:

❧ DOES THE DOCTOR TAKE X-RAYS OF THEIR PATIENTS? THOUGH NOT ALL CHIROPRACTIC TECHNIQUES REQUIRE THE USE OF X-RAY, SEEING THE SPINE ON X-RAY ELIMINATES GUESSWORK AND GIVES AN INDICATION OF HOW THOROUGH THE CHIROPRACTOR IS.

- ♛ DO THEY CARE FOR CHILDREN? THIS IS A CLUE TO HOW PASSIONATE THE CHIROPRACTOR IS ABOUT THEIR LIFE'S WORK.

- ♛ DO THEY RECOMMEND REGULAR LIFETIME SPINAL CARE? IF NOT, HE OR SHE ONLY PROVIDES SHORT-TERM PAIN RELIEF. YOU ARE LOOKING FOR A CHIROPRACTOR WHO ADVOCATES SPINAL CORRECTION <u>AND</u> LONG-TERM WELLNESS, NOT JUST PAIN RELIEF. THIS REGULAR CARE IS VITAL IN KEEPING YOUR NERVOUS SYSTEM FUNCTIONING AT ITS OPTIMUM.

- ♛ HOW LONG DO OFFICE VISITS GENERALLY TAKE? A TYPICAL ROUTINE VISIT SHOULD TAKE ONLY 10-20 MINUTES.

- ♛ DO THEY HAVE A FAMILY PLAN? A DEVOTED CORRECTIVE/ WELLNESS CARE CHIROPRACTOR WILL WANT TO CHECK YOUR WHOLE FAMILY. THEY WILL ALSO HAVE FAMILY PLANS AVAILABLE TO MAKE IT AFFORDABLE TO DO SO.

- ♛ ASK IF THE DOCTOR HAS EXPERIENCE WORKING WITH YOUR TYPE OF HEALTH PROBLEM (IF YOU HAVE ONE).

Take the time to find the best chiropractor in your area. It is worth the time to find a great chiropractor who will thoroughly examine your family's spines and start care quickly to help you begin enjoying health and healing.

Lord, thank you for designing my body to heal itself. Thank you that I do not have to be afraid of every germ I am exposed to, but that You have given my body the ability to fight sickness and disease. Help me to do everything I can to maintain a strong immune system and stay healthy. I want to be fully available for the kingdom work You planned for me. You are worthy of my praise! Amen.

Becoming a Healthier You
– In Review

- ♛ MODERN MEDICINE IS BASED ON THE GERM THEORY OF DISEASE — THAT SICKNESS AND DISEASE ARE THE RESULT OF COMING IN CONTACT WITH GERMS SUCH AS BACTERIA OR A VIRUS.

- ♛ THE TRUE CAUSE OF SICKNESS IS INTERFERENCE WITH THE BODY'S ABILITY TO HEAL. SUBLUXATIONS BLOCK PROPER NERVE FLOW THROUGH THE BODY, DECREASING YOUR IMMUNE RESISTANCE AND RESULTING IN SICKNESS.

- ♛ DRUGS AND SURGERY DO NOT REMOVE INTERFERENCE; THEY MAY REMOVE SYMPTOMS AND CAN ACTUALLY MAKE YOU SICKER.

- ♛ SUBLUXATIONS IN THE SPINE ARE ONE OF THE BIGGEST CAUSES OF LOWERED IMMUNITY. IN ADDITION, A POOR DIET, LACK OF EXERCISE, LACK OF SLEEP AND HIGH STRESS LEVELS WILL ALSO LOWER YOUR IMMUNITY AND MAKE YOU MORE SUSCEPTIBLE TO SICKNESS.

- ♛ THE ART AND SCIENCE OF CHIROPRACTIC HAS PROGRESSED WITH ADVANCED DIAGNOSTIC PROCEDURES, SOPHISTICATED EQUIPMENT AND SCIENTIFIC RESEARCH.

- ♛ GETTING YOUR SPINE ADJUSTED IS A SIMPLE, COMFORTABLE PROCEDURE THAT ONLY TAKES A FEW MINUTES EACH VISIT.

- ♛ CHIROPRACTIC CARE IS A LIFE-LONG APPROACH TO HEALTH AND WELL BEING. A HEALTHY SPINE MEANS A HEALTHIER YOU.

* A SECONDARY BENEFIT OF CHIROPRACTIC CARE IS HOW IT LOWERS THE COST OF HEALTH CARE IN GENERAL.

* WHEN YOU SEARCH FOR A CHIROPRACTOR, THE GOAL IS TO FIND THE BEST IN YOUR AREA.

Were you taught that sickness is "caught" by exposure to germs? Now that you know more about how your immune system works, do you have a new perspective on why people get sick? _____

_____

_____

_____

Does "feeling good" mean that you are experiencing good health? Why not? _____

_____

_____

_____

_____

What is the true cause of sickness and disease? (See Myth #2.)

_____

_____

_____

Do drugs, surgery and doctors make people well, or do they too often only treat symptoms?_____

_____

_____

_____

Would you like to decrease your health care expenses?_____

_____

_____

_____

If you are not currently under chiropractic care, follow the steps outlined in the chapter to find the most qualified chiropractic office in your area. _____

_____

_____

_____

Notes: _____

_____

_____

_____

_____

_____

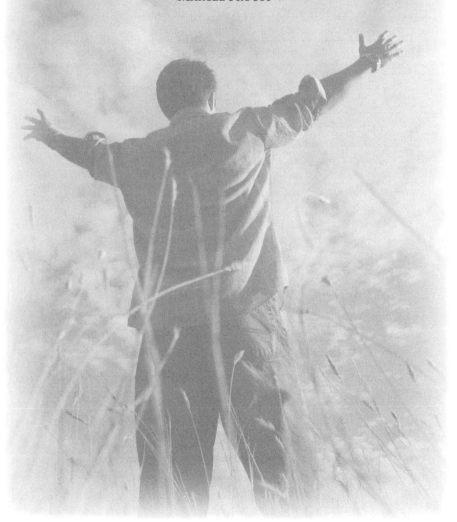

Illness is the doctor to whom we pay most heed;
to kindness, to knowledge, we make promise only;
pain we obey.

— ❧ —

MARCEL PROUST

Chapter Twenty-One

Why Christians Get Sick

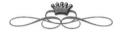

IT IS AN UNFORTUNATE FACT that Christians get sick just as often as non-Christians but this is not God's will for His children. After seeing thousands of my own patients walking in divine health and healing, you will never convince me that it is God's will or desire for His people to be sick and suffering. How can we believe that His good plans include suffering an agonizing, prolonged death from cancer or that it would be in His will for a forty-year-old father of three small children to drop over dead of a massive heart attack?

Scripture does record an infirmity that God allowed in order to bring glory to his name in 1 John 9; however, I believe that these circumstances are very rare. The kind of sickness that I can unequivocally say is *not* within God's will for His people are the Top Ten Killers – primarily because they are all avoidable. Regardless of this fact, virtually every person (78 percent) in the United States as well as other developed countries will die from one of the top ten. This is most definitely *not* God's will for you!

So why do Christians get sick? In addition to the other reasons already discussed in previous chapters, here are five possible reasons:

1.   Lack of Knowledge

Some Christians are simply unaware of how to take proper care of their bodies to achieve divine health.

2.   Lack of Self Discipline

This group of Christians knows what they should be doing to walk in better health but lacks the self discipline to carry it out in daily living. In my opinion, most unhealthy Christians fit into this category. Our culture is health-minded; even if everyone is not walking the walk, there are enough people talking the talk that few of us can claim total ignorance. Just take a look at all of the health and fitness books and magazines that are available in the grocery checkout line and at your local bookstore.

> *It is an unfortunate fact that Christians get sick just as often as non-Christians.*

I can sympathize with Christians who have a difficult time disciplining themselves because I know that very few people want to be lazy when it comes to their health, and of course everyone wants to look better on the outside. The truth remains, however, that our bodies are the temple of the Holy Spirit and we have a *spiritual mandate* to care for that temple.[52]

Christians who lack self discipline are forced to rely on "Hope Management."

Very often Christians who lack self discipline in the area of health are forced to rely on "Hope Management." They simply hope that sickness and disease will not come their way and that all their bad habits (poor food choices, weight gain, lack of exercise, overuse of prescription and over-the-counter drugs, etc.) will never catch up to them.

3. Unforgiveness

It has been said that the bitterness caused by unforgiveness is like drinking poison and hoping that someone else dies. When we choose not to forgive God or someone who has wronged us we intentionally walk into an unending cycle of stress, anger, worry and torment. Over time, these negative emotions open the door for sickness to walk right in and destroy our health and lives. Choose to forgive and release those who have wronged you in the same way Christ freely forgives you, and experience the peace and ensuing good health that forgiveness brings.

4. The Violation of God's Natural Laws

There is a cause/effect relationship in the spiritual realm that not many Christians seem aware of or concerned about.

---

52   "Or do you not know that your body is a temple of the Holy Spirit who is in you, whom you have from God, and that you are not your own?" 1 Corinthians 6:19

In his book *Why Christians Get Sick,* Dr. George H. Malkmus addresses the result of violating God's natural laws:

> In 1 Corinthians 3:16-19 we read, "Know ye not that ye are the temple of God, and that the spirit of God dwelleth in you? If any man defile the temple of God, him shall God destroy; for the temple of God is holy, which temple ye are."
>
> These scriptures puzzled me for many years. It was not until I personally had physical problems, which resulted in my studying how the body functions and in learning the importance of proper nutrition and vigorous exercise, that my eyes were opened to what the Bible was teaching here in 1 Corinthians 3:16-18.
>
> There is additional teaching on this subject in 1 Corinthians 6:19-20: "What, know ye not that your body is the temple of the Holy Ghost which is in you, which ye have of God, and ye are not your own? For ye are bought with a price: therefore glorify God in your body, and in your spirit, which are God's."
>
> Clearly, the Bible teaches that *the Christian's body is not his own.... it belongs to God!* If a Christian fails to care properly for his body, *God will destroy that body!* Let's read that scripture again... *"If any man defile* ('make unclean with something unpleasant or contaminating' Webster) *the temple of God, him shall God destroy."* (1 Corinthians 3:17 KJV) [53]

---

53   Malkmus, Dr. George H. (1995). <u>Why Christians Get Sick</u> (16th ed.). Shippensburg, PA: Destiny Image Publishers, Inc.

Dr. Malkmus came to believe that violating God's natural laws caused over 90 percent of all sickness that Christians experience. People are simply not properly caring for and honoring their bodies as God's holy dwelling place.

5. *Demonic Influences*

Though I am no expert in this area I am convinced that we can become sick when we open doors to demonic influence in our lives through the use of illegal drugs, satanic worship, unrighteous living, etc. Demonic influence, oppression and demonic possession are real and occur in our world today.

Thankfully, we serve a God who is greater than the demonic powers of this world![54] The Lord Jesus is also eager to forgive and restore us when we turn from our sinful ways and become obedient to His word.[55] If you are involved in sinful behaviors that are opening the door to demonic influences, seek help from your local church congregation and trust that the power of Jesus' blood will bring deliverance in your life.

> *You have rights and privileges as a child of God.*

If you are a Christian you have rights and privileges as a child of God. One of them is to walk in divine health with the help and empowerment of the Holy Spirit. Start walking in all of God's promises today. He has provided a body built for

---

54   "You, dear children, are from God and have overcome them, because the one who is in you is greater than the one who is in the world." 1 John 4:4

55   "If we confess our sins, he is faithful and just and will forgive us our sins and purify us from all unrighteousness." 1 John 1:9

health and healing and it is your duty as a Christian to care for the vessel that He inhabits. Ask the Holy Spirit to guide and direct you as you become a healthier person spiritually, emotionally and physically.

> L ord, I know that it must grieve you to see so many of your children suffering from pain and disease. Thank you that you have provided a better way for me to live. I give your Holy Spirit permission to point out areas of my life where I am not living as you desire. Give me strength and the self discipline to overcome my areas of weakness. Thank you that you are walking with me on this journey to divine health and healing. I rebuke sickness and disease in my life and my family today and claim the good health that you desire for me. I pray this in Jesus' name. Amen.

Why Christians Get Sick
– In Review

- ♛ CHRISTIANS GET SICK AS OFTEN AS NON-CHRISTIANS DO.

- ♛ IT IS NOT GOD'S WILL FOR CHRISTIANS TO SUFFER AND DIE FROM THE TOP TEN KILLERS.

- ♛ IN ADDITION TO POOR DIETS, LACK OF EXERCISE AND EXPOSURE TO TOXIC CHEMICALS, THERE ARE A FEW OTHER POSSIBLE REASONS THAT CHRISTIANS GET SICK. THEY ARE:

  1. LACK OF KNOWLEDGE

  2. LACK OF SELF DISCIPLINE

  3. UNFORGIVENESS

  4. THE VIOLATION OF GOD'S NATURAL LAWS

  5. DEMONIC INFLUENCES

- ♛ CHRISTIANS HAVE RIGHTS AND PRIVILEGES AS CHILDREN OF GOD.

- ♛ ONE PRIVILEGE IS THE ABILITY TO WALK IN DIVINE HEALTH.

- ♛ GOD HAS PROVIDED BODIES CAPABLE OF DIVINE HEALTH AND HEALING AND IT IS OUR RESPONSIBILITY TO LIVE IN A WAY THAT PROMOTES DIVINE HEALTH AND HEALING.

As a Christian, are you troubled by how many of our brothers and sisters are struggling with sickness and disease? Does this seem consistent with what you believe about God's will for His people? _____

_____

_____

Are you walking in the level of divine health that you know God desires for you?_____

_____

_____

If not, why? Do you lack knowledge? Do you lack self discipline? Do any other reasons for sickness from the list in this chapter apply to you?_____

_____

_____

_____

What can you do to be rid of this hindrance to divine health?

_____

_____

_____

Have you claimed divine health and healing as your right as a child of God? Take a moment right now and ask God to reveal to you the root of any health issues. Ask for the strength, wisdom and discipline to overcome them._____

_____

_____

_____

Notes: _____

_____

_____

_____

_____

_____

_____

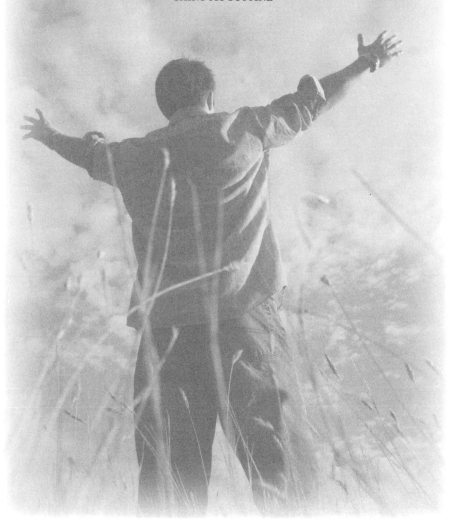

Faith is to believe what you do not see;
the reward of this faith is to see
what you believe.

SAINT AUGUSTINE

Chapter Twenty-Two

The Power of Faith and Prayer

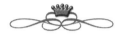

TWO VITAL COMPONENTS of staying "Fit for the King" are fundamentals of the Christian walk. They are faith and prayer. Hebrews 11:6 is very clear that "…. without faith it is impossible to please God, because anyone who comes to him must believe that he exists and that he rewards those who earnestly seek him." Likewise, Ephesians 6:18 stresses the importance of prayer: "And pray in the Spirit on all occasions with all kinds of prayers and requests. With this in mind, be alert and always keep on praying for all the saints." Have no doubt that God is on your side and desires that you live an abundant, healthy, joyful life!

Increasing your faith in God's goodness and faithfulness is one way that Christian's can stay strong and healthy.

> *A simple way to increase your faith is to meditate on scriptures that remind you of God's desire to bless his people.*

A very simple way to increase your faith and promote physical, emotional and spiritual health is to meditate on scriptures that remind you of God's desire to bless his people. Here are a few of my favorite scriptures that speak to His desire to prosper, bless, and heal:

Worship the Lord your God, and his blessing will be on your food and water. I will take away sickness from among you, and none will miscarry or be barren in your land. I will give you a full life span. Exodus 23:25-26

You will be blessed more than any other people; none of your men or women will be childless, nor any of your livestock without young. The Lord will keep you free from every disease. He will not inflict on you the horrible diseases you knew in Egypt, but he will inflict them on all who hate you. Deuteronomy 7:14-15

If you fully obey the Lord your God and carefully follow all his commands I give you today, the Lord your God will set you high above all the nations on earth. All these blessings will come upon you and accompany you if you obey the Lord your God: You will be blessed in the city and blessed in the country. The fruit of your womb will be blessed, and the crops of your land and the young of your livestock—the calves of your herds and the lambs of your flocks. Your basket and your kneading trough will be blessed. You will be blessed when you come in and blessed when you go out. The Lord will grant that the

> *They will come at you from one direction but flee from you in seven.*

enemies who rise up against you will be defeated before you. They will come at you from one direction but flee from you in seven. The Lord will send a blessing on your barns and on everything you put your hand to. The Lord your God will bless you in the land he is giving you. The Lord will establish you as his holy people, as he promised you on oath, if you keep the commands of the Lord your God and walk in his ways. Then all the peoples on earth will see that you are called by the name of the Lord, and they will fear you. The Lord will grant you abundant prosperity—in the fruit of your womb, the young of your livestock and the crops of your ground—in the land he swore to your forefathers to give you. The Lord will open the heavens, the storehouse of his bounty, to send rain on your land in season and to bless all the work of your hands. You will lend to many nations but will borrow from none. The Lord will make you the head, not the tail. If you pay attention to the commands of the Lord your God that I give you this day and carefully follow them, you will always be at the top, never at the bottom. Do not turn aside from any of the commands I give you today, to the right or to the left, following other gods and serving them. Deuteronomy 28:1-14

"For I know the plans I have for you," declares the Lord, "plans to prosper you and not to harm you, plans to give you hope and a future." Jeremiah 29:11

The thief comes only to steal and kill and destroy; I have come that they may have life, and have it to the full. John 10:10

> *Many Christians do not realize the importance of asking God in prayer to protect their health.*
>
> ♛

Letting these truths soak into your hearts and mind requires that you slow down and listen for God's still, small voice confirming His word to your spirit. The Holy Spirit stands ready to speak to you in very personal ways if you will take the time to sit quietly in His presence and spend time meditating on His word. As you read of His eagerness to bless and prosper you, your faith will increase and so will your health!

Our response to the voice of God through scripture and meditation is worship, prayer, praise and gratitude. You may have never considered that these responses are actually a very vital part of your physical healthcare routine, but they are too important to be overlooked! Specifically, I believe that many Christians do not realize the importance of asking God in prayer to protect their health and the health of those they love.

In her wonderful book *Protecting Your Family in Dangerous Times,* Kelly Copeland Kutz, daughter of Kenneth and Gloria Copeland, shows how to have absolute certainty of divine protection:

> Here is an absolute guarantee: *There is no more certain place to be than in the presence of God. And when I say certain, I mean safe, secure and assured.* You can count on it. Even if the Lord prompts you to go minister to someone in a hospital filled with deadly, contagious diseases, you can go with confidence and peace. Why? Be-

cause you know you are walking in God's presence, and in that divine presence is certain, supernatural protection.

Whenever the Lord says with great certainty in His Word that you can possess something, it should be very difficult for the devil to take that promise away from you. On the other hand, it may be harder for you to be confident if you are praying for something that isn't specifically promised in the Word. In that case, you need a strong inner knowing from the Holy Spirit that the petition you have asked for is yours to claim.

You are a covenant person. Therefore, you should be confident that God will perform His promise of protection for you as you stand in His presence by faith.[56]

I encourage you to pick up a copy of Kelly's book and give it serious consideration. The wisdom she imparts will prevent calamity and increase your faith in God's protection of your family. Psalm 91:7-8 says that, "A thousand may fall at your side, ten thousand at your right hand, but it will not come near you. You will only observe with your eyes and see the punishment of the wicked."

There is strong biblical precedent for praying for safety and protection over ourselves and our loved ones. In the Old Testament, God instructed the Israelites to place the blood of a spotless

There is strong biblical precedent for praying for safety and protection.

---

56   Kutz, Kelly Copeland (2003). <u>Protecting Your Family in Dangerous Times</u> Tulsa, OK: Harrison House

lamb around the doorposts of their home. When they obeyed, the angel of death would pass over their household.[57] As New Testament believers we are covered with the precious blood of Jesus. Every day my wife and I plead the blood of Jesus over us, our children, our personal property and our businesses. We trust God and believe in His divine protection over everything and everyone we name in prayer.

You have the same right and privilege as a believer of Jesus Christ! Pray daily over your own health, your spouse, your family and friends. I believe that these prayers of faith create a force field around you spiritually that our enemy, Satan, and his demonic angels are unable to penetrate. In addition, our prayers release angels who stand by to guard and protect us.

This is how my wife, Karen, and I pray every day: "We plead the blood of Jesus over John, Karen, Jonathan and Kayla (our children). We thank you, Lord, for perfect health and wholeness in our bodies. We plead your blood over our property, our businesses, our patients, our employees and their families. We ask you to release angels to guard over us, protect us, minister to us and open doors for us. Thank you for giving us favor everywhere we turn and for prospering the work of our hands.

---

57 "Tell the whole community of Israel that on the tenth day of this month each man is to take a lamb for his family, one for each household. The animals you choose must be year-old males without defect, and you may take them from the sheep or the goats. Take care of them until the fourteenth day of the month, when all the people of the community of Israel must slaughter them at twilight. On that same night I will pass through Egypt and strike down every firstborn—both men and animals—and I will bring judgment on all the gods of Egypt. I am the Lord. The blood will be a sign for you on the houses where you are; and when I see the blood, I will pass over you. No destructive plague will touch you when I strike Egypt." Exodus 12:3,5&6

Thank you for protecting us from calamity. Give us wisdom to make good choices and order all of our steps today. Amen."

As you meditate on scripture and plead the blood of Jesus over your life, you will increasingly have "the mind of Christ" referred to in 1 Corinthians 2:16.[58] Having your focus on the Lord will naturally cause you to make wise decisions that will guard your health and your life, but this protection requires that you are completely surrendered to His leading and obedient to His will.

When Christians lack faith they open the door for the enemy to walk in and steal their health.

The word of God tells us Satan roams about like a hungry, roaring lion.[59] He is looking for people who are not living under the protective blood of Jesus. When Christians lack faith, do not pray for protection, walk in disobedience to God's will or do not take proper care of their physical bodies they open the door for the enemy to walk in and steal their health. In essence, they turn away from the divine protection Jesus bought with His blood.

You have been given wonderful privileges as the son or daughter of the King. Enjoy divine health and healing by claiming every promise that God made to you. Meditate on His word, pray daily over yourself and your family and enjoy the peace of knowing that God is watching and guarding over you.

---

58   "For who has known the mind of the Lord that he may instruct him? But we have the mind of Christ." 1 Corinthians 2:16

59   "Be self-controlled and alert. Your enemy the devil prowls around like a roaring lion looking for someone to devour." 1 Peter 5:8

In righteousness you will be established: tyranny will be far from you; you will have nothing to fear. Terror will be far removed; it will not come near you. If anyone does attack you, it will not be my doing; whoever attacks you will surrender to you. No weapon forged against you will prevail, and you will refute every tongue that accuses you. This is the heritage of the servants of the Lord, and this is their vindication from me,' declares the Lord. Isaiah 54:14, 15&17

He who dwells in the shelter of the Most High will rest in the shadow of the Almighty. I will say of the Lord, "He is my refuge and my fortress, my God, in whom I trust." Surely he will save you from the fowler's snare and from the deadly pestilence. He will cover you with his feathers, and under his wings you will find refuge; his faithfulness will be your shield and rampart. You will not fear the terror of night, nor the arrow that flies by day, nor the pestilence that stalks in the darkness, nor the plague that destroys at midday. A thousand may fall at your side, ten thousand at your right hand, but it will not come near you. You will only observe with your eyes and see the punishment of the wicked. Psalm 91:1-8

God honors His word and loves His people. Experience all of the blessings that Jesus purchased for you on the cross and enjoy the life of whole, health and healing that He desires for you.

Thank you, Lord, that you desire to bless and prosper me in every way. Thank you that you shed your blood to purchase every good thing that I need. Help me to spend more time meditating on your goodness and increase my faith. As I read your word, please speak to me personally and remind me of your goodness. Help me to be more diligent in praying for myself and my loved ones. Thank you that you release your angels to guard and protect me. I rebuke Satan's attacks on my life and health in the name of Jesus, and I claim every good thing that you bought for me on the cross. Amen.

The Power of Faith and Prayer – In Review

- FAITH AND PRAYER ARE FUNDAMENTALS OF THE CHRISTIAN LIFE AND ARE VITALLY IMPORTANT TO DIVINE HEALTH AND HEALING.

- GOD'S PLANS FOR HIS CHILDREN ARE GOOD. HE DESIRES THAT EVERY CHRISTIAN LIVES AN ABUNDANT, HEALTHY, JOYFUL LIFE.

- A VERY SIMPLE WAY TO INCREASE YOUR FAITH AND PROMOTE PHYSICAL, EMOTIONAL AND SPIRITUAL HEALTH IS TO MEDITATE ON SCRIPTURES THAT REMIND YOU OF GOD'S DESIRE TO BLESS HIS PEOPLE.

- THE HOLY SPIRIT STANDS READY TO SPEAK TO YOU IN VERY PERSONAL WAYS IF YOU WILL TAKE THE TIME TO SIT QUIETLY IN HIS PRESENCE WITH THE WORD OF GOD OPEN BEFORE YOU.

- MANY CHRISTIANS DO NOT REALIZE THE IMPORTANCE OF ASKING GOD IN PRAYER TO PROTECT THEIR HEALTH AND THE HEALTH OF THOSE THEY LOVE.

- PLEAD THE BLOOD OF JESUS DAILY OVER YOUR OWN HEALTH, YOUR SPOUSE, YOUR FAMILY AND FRIENDS.

- THESE PRAYERS OF FAITH CREATE A FORCE FIELD AROUND YOU SPIRITUALLY THAT OUR ENEMY, SATAN, AND HIS DEMONIC ANGELS ARE UNABLE TO PENETRATE. IN ADDITION, OUR PRAYERS RELEASE ANGELS WHO STAND BY TO GUARD AND PROTECT US.

- AS YOU MEDITATE ON SCRIPTURE AND PLEAD THE BLOOD OF JESUS OVER YOUR LIFE, YOU WILL INCREASINGLY HAVE "THE MIND OF CHRIST."

✦ WHEN CHRISTIANS LACK FAITH, DO NOT PRAY FOR PROTECTION AND WALK IN DISOBEDIENCE TO GOD'S WILL, THEY OPEN THE DOOR FOR THE ENEMY TO WALK IN AND STEAL THEIR HEALTH.

✦ CHRISTIANS WHO LEAN ON THE POWER OF FAITH AND PRAYER HAVE PEACE THAT GOD IS GUARDING AND PROTECTING THEIR HEALTH AND LIFE.

Do you have a personal devotional time every day where you meditate on the word of God and listen for His spirit to speak to you? If not, determine to make a commitment to this practice and record when and where you will spend this quiet time with the Lord. _____

_____

_____

_____

Have you experienced God's faithfulness in a personal way in your life? Record some of the things God has done for you in the past and consider keeping a journal of His faithfulness in your own life. _____

_____

_____

_____

_____

Has it ever occurred to you to plead the blood of Jesus over your life and your loved ones before? _____

_____

_____

Commit to praying this life-changing prayer every day. List the people and things that you will include in this prayer (family members, friends, employers, property, etc.)_____

_____

_____

_____

Pause and ask God to give you "the mind of Christ" as you make decisions about your health going forward. _____

_____

_____

_____

Are there any areas of disobedience in your life right now that might be opening a door for Satan to enter and steal your health? _____

_____

_____

_____

What do you need to do to close those doors and walk in obedience to God's will?_____

_____

_____

_____

Notes: _____

_____

_____

_____

_____

_____

_____

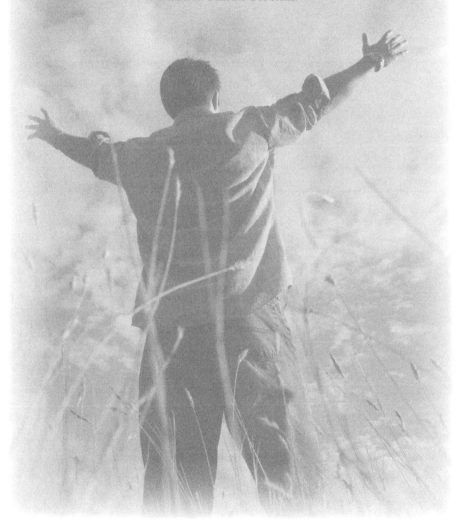

*Half the modern drugs could well be
thrown out of the window,
except that the birds might eat them.*

———❧———

MARTIN HENRY FISCHER

Chapter Twenty-Three

A Prescription for Healing

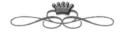

WE HAVE MADE some important discoveries and come to some wonderful conclusions. God made your body to walk in divine health and healing. It is not His will for you to be sick, to suffer from disease, or to die early from one of the Top Ten Killers. This is all wonderful news!

But what if this information is new to you and you have already received a frightening diagnosis? Is all hope lost? Absolutely not! God is still in the miracle-working business and longs to *partner with you* toward the goal of divine health and healing. There are many steps you can take right now to make healing a strong possibility in your life and body.

It is never too late to become a healthier you. Your body can and will respond to true "healthcare." Though it may not bounce back as quickly as it did when you were younger, even a 20-30 percent improvement in your physical health can make a profound difference. In God's health economy, a little effort pays big dividends. You can still add life to your years and years to your life!

Some of you have already received a frightening diagnosis of diabetes, cancer, heart disease, blocked arteries, chronic fatigue syndrome or multiple sclerosis. Others are battling COPD (chronic obstructive pulmonary disease – a serious lung condition), brain tumors, Irritable Bowel Syndrome, prostatitis or any of several dozen other serious and life threatening diseases or disorders. I want to give you ten steps that will move you toward divine health and healing immediately. Any one of them can be started *today* to ensure that *tomorrow* is a healthier, more joyful day.

Ten Steps for Healing

1. *Believe Psalm 112:6-8 for your life.*

   "Surely he will never be shaken; a righteous man will be remembered forever. He will have no fear of bad news; his heart is steadfast, trusting in the Lord. His heart is secure, he will have no fear; in the end he will look in triumph on his foes."

   You are a child of God and no matter what circumstances you face, nothing can change that fact! I encourage you to write down this verse and the ones that follow and post them in places in your home where you will see them many times each day. They will bring peace to your heart and will increase your faith as you meditate on them.

2. *Spend time in prayer.*

This seems like a trite answer because many of us quickly rush to pray when we face difficult circumstances. Unfortunately, our common plea is, "God, help me!" and we end with that. No, the kind of prayer I encourage you to engage in is a conversation with God. Ask Him to show you why you became sick. Ask Him to reveal what changes you need to make. Bare your heart to Him. If you are angry about your diagnosis, tell Him! (He knows your every thought before a word is on your tongue anyway![60]) God longs to speak to you in deeply personal ways. It is His desire to redeem every good thing He can out of every circumstance you face. Many people who face life-threatening diagnoses are actually thankful for the renewed intimacy with God that develops as a result. Pour your heart out to your loving Heavenly Father often, and seek His will as you determine how to best battle your health condition.

3. *Rally the troops.*

Inform your closest, most faith-filled friends about the health situation you are facing. You are looking for spiritual giants who will agree with you for total and complete healing. I like to think of this group of people as a "prayer corral" with all of their wagons circled and you in the middle, safe and protected. Do not include anyone in the corral who you feel will not have strong faith to believe for your full healing. No unbelief allowed! Pray the words of Matthew 18:18-19 often and with courage:

---

60   " Before a word is on my tongue you know it completely, O LORD." Psalm 139:4

"I tell you the truth, whatever you bind on earth will be bound in heaven, and whatever you loose on earth will be loosed in heaven. Again, I tell you that if two of you on earth agree about anything you ask for, it will be done for you by my Father in heaven."

4. *Be anointed for healing.*

James 5:14-16 says, "Is any one of you sick? He should call the elders of the church to pray over him and anoint him with oil in the name of the Lord. And the prayer offered in faith will make the sick person well; the Lord will raise him up. If he has sinned, he will be forgiven. Therefore confess your sins to each other and pray for each other so that you may be healed. The prayer of a righteous man is powerful and effective."

We have this right and privilege as believers. What an awesome experience to have faith-filled elders lay their hands on you and anoint you for healing!

5. *Take your spiritual medicine.*

Nothing is more encouraging than spending some quiet time in the word of God when you are facing threatening circumstances and health problems. There are many passages and Bible stories that will fill you with hope and increase your faith for healing. Following are some healing scriptures that will get you started.[61] Gloria Copeland suggests in her healing school that you take scripture like

Take scripture like medicine, three times per day.

---

61   Consider getting a copy of Kenneth and Gloria Copeland's book <u>Healing Promises</u>. It is an excellent resource full of healing scriptures. You can order their book online at: www.kcm.org.

medicine, three times per day, reading them aloud and confessing them in full faith, believing that every word is true.

Healing Scriptures

Exodus 23:25

[25] Worship the Lord your God, and his blessing will be on your food and water. I will take away sickness from among you....

Psalm 91:9-10

[9] If you make the Most High your dwelling—
even the Lord, who is my refuge-

[10] then no harm will befall you,
no disaster will come near your tent.

Psalm 91:14-16

[14] "Because he loves me," says the Lord, "I will rescue him;
I will protect him, for he acknowledges my name.

[15] He will call upon me, and I will answer him;
I will be with him in trouble,
I will deliver him and honor him.

[16] With long life will I satisfy him
and show him my salvation."

Psalm 103

[1] Praise the Lord, O my soul;
all my inmost being, praise his holy name.

² Praise the Lord, O my soul,
    and forget not all his benefits-

³ who forgives all your sins
    and heals all your diseases,

⁴ who redeems your life from the pit
    and crowns you with love and compassion,

⁵ who satisfies your desires with good things
    so that your youth is renewed like the eagle's.

Psalm 107:19-21

¹⁹ Then they cried to the Lord in their trouble,
    and he saved them from their distress.

²⁰ He sent forth his word and healed them;
    he rescued them from the grave.

²¹ Let them give thanks to the Lord for his unfailing love
    and his wonderful deeds for men.

Psalm 112:6-8

⁶ Surely he will never be shaken;
    a righteous man will be remembered forever.

⁷ He will have no fear of bad news;
    his heart is steadfast, trusting in the Lord.

⁸ His heart is secure, he will have no fear;
    in the end he will look in triumph on his foes.

Psalm 118:17

¹⁷ I will not die but live,
    and will proclaim what the Lord has done.

Proverbs 4:20-24

[20] My son, pay attention to what I say;
   listen closely to my words.

[21] Do not let them out of your sight,
   keep them within your heart;

[22] for they are life to those who find them
   and health to a man's whole body.

[23] Above all else, guard your heart,
   for it is the wellspring of life.

[24] Put away perversity from your mouth;
   keep corrupt talk far from your lips

Isaiah 40:28-31

[28] Do you not know?
   Have you not heard?
   The Lord is the everlasting God,
   the Creator of the ends of the earth.
   He will not grow tired or weary,
   and his understanding no one can fathom.

[29] He gives strength to the weary
   and increases the power of the weak.

[30] Even youths grow tired and weary,
   and young men stumble and fall;

[31] but those who hope in the Lord
   will renew their strength.
   They will soar on wings like eagles;
   they will run and not grow weary,
   they will walk and not be faint.

Isaiah 41:10

[10] So do not fear, for I am with you;
    do not be dismayed, for I am your God.
    I will strengthen you and help you;
    I will uphold you with my righteous right hand.

Isaiah 53:4-5

[4] Surely he took up our infirmities
    and carried our sorrows,
    yet we considered him stricken by God,
    smitten by him, and afflicted.

[5] But he was pierced for our transgressions,
    he was crushed for our iniquities;
    the punishment that brought us peace was upon him,
    and by his wounds we are healed.

Isaiah 54:17

[17] "....no weapon forged against you will prevail,
    and you will refute every tongue that accuses you.
    This is the heritage of the servants of the Lord,
    and this is their vindication from me,"
    declares the Lord.

Jeremiah 30:17

[17] But I will restore you to health
    and heal your wounds,'
    declares the Lord,
    'because you are called an outcast,
    Zion for whom no one cares.'

Nahum 1:9

⁹ Whatever they plot against the Lord
  he will bring to an end;
    trouble will not come a second time.

Malachi 4:2

² But for you who revere my name, the sun of righteousness will rise with healing in its wings. And you will go out and leap like calves released from the stall.

Matthew 4:23-24

²³Jesus went throughout Galilee, teaching in their synagogues, preaching the good news of the kingdom, and healing every disease and sickness among the people. ²⁴News about him spread all over Syria, and people brought to him all who were ill with various diseases, those suffering severe pain, the demon-possessed, those having seizures, and the paralyzed, and he healed them.

Matthew 8:2-3

²A man with leprosy came and knelt before him and said, "Lord, if you are willing, you can make me clean."

³Jesus reached out his hand and touched the man. "I am willing," he said. "Be clean!" Immediately he was cured of his leprosy.

Matthew 8:13

¹³Then Jesus said to the centurion, "Go! It will be done just as you believed it would." And his servant was healed at that very hour.

Matthew 8:16-17

[16]When evening came, many who were demon-possessed were brought to him, and he drove out the spirits with a word and healed all the sick. [17]This was to fulfill what was spoken through the prophet Isaiah:

"He took up our infirmities and carried our diseases."

Matthew 9:20-22

[20]Just then a woman who had been subject to bleeding for twelve years came up behind him and touched the edge of his cloak. [21]She said to herself, "If I only touch his cloak, I will be healed."

[22]Jesus turned and saw her. "Take heart, daughter," he said, "your faith has healed you." And the woman was healed from that moment.

Matthew 9:35

[35]Jesus went through all the towns and villages, teaching in their synagogues, preaching the good news of the kingdom and healing every disease and sickness.

Matthew 12:13

[13]Then he said to the man, "Stretch out your hand." So he stretched it out and it was completely restored, just as sound as the other.

Matthew 15:30-31

[30]Great crowds came to him, bringing the lame, the blind, the crippled, the mute and many others, and laid them at his feet; and he healed them. [31]The people were amazed

when they saw the mute speaking, the crippled made well, the lame walking and the blind seeing. And they praised the God of Israel.

Matthew 18:18-19

[18]"I tell you the truth, whatever you bind on earth will be bound in heaven, and whatever you loose on earth will be loosed in heaven.

[19]"Again, I tell you that if two of you on earth agree about anything you ask for, it will be done for you by my Father in heaven.

Matthew 20:32-34

[32]Jesus stopped and called them. "What do you want me to do for you?" he asked.

[33]"Lord," they answered, "we want our sight."

[34]Jesus had compassion on them and touched their eyes. Immediately they received their sight and followed him.

Matthew 21:21

[21]Jesus replied, "I tell you the truth, if you have faith and do not doubt, not only can you do what was done to the fig tree, but also you can say to this mountain, 'Go, throw yourself into the sea,' and it will be done.

Mark 1:40-42

[40]A man with leprosy came to him and begged him on his knees, "If you are willing, you can make me clean."

⁴¹Filled with compassion, Jesus reached out his hand and touched the man. "I am willing," he said. "Be clean!" ⁴²Immediately the leprosy left him and he was cured.

Mark 6:7, 12-13

⁷Calling the Twelve to him, he sent them out two by two and gave them authority over evil spirits. ¹²They went out and preached that people should repent. ¹³They drove out many demons and anointed many sick people with oil and healed them.

Mark 11:22-24

²²"Have faith in God," Jesus answered. ²³"I tell you the truth, if anyone says to this mountain, 'Go, throw yourself into the sea,' and does not doubt in his heart but believes that what he says will happen, it will be done for him. ²⁴Therefore I tell you, whatever you ask for in prayer, believe that you have received it, and it will be yours.

Luke 4:40

⁴⁰When the sun was setting, the people brought to Jesus all who had various kinds of sickness, and laying his hands on each one, he healed them.

Luke 6:17-19

¹⁷He went down with them and stood on a level place. A large crowd of his disciples was there and a great number of people from all over Judea, from Jerusalem, and from the coast of Tyre and Sidon, ¹⁸who had come to hear him and to be healed of their diseases. Those troubled by evil spirits

were cured, [19]and the people all tried to touch him, because power was coming from him and healing them all.

Luke 7:14-15

[14]Then he went up and touched the coffin, and those carrying it stood still. He said, "Young man, I say to you, get up!" [15]The dead man sat up and began to talk, and Jesus gave him back to his mother.

Luke 9:1-2,6

[1]When Jesus had called the Twelve together, he gave them power and authority to drive out all demons and to cure diseases, [2]and he sent them out to preach the kingdom of God and to heal the sick. [6]So they set out and went from village to village, preaching the gospel and healing people everywhere.

Luke 13:10-14

[10]On a Sabbath Jesus was teaching in one of the synagogues, [11]and a woman was there who had been crippled by a spirit for eighteen years. She was bent over and could not straighten up at all. [12]When Jesus saw her, he called her forward and said to her, "Woman, you are set free from your infirmity." [13]Then he put his hands on her, and immediately she straightened up and praised God.

John 10:10

[10]The thief comes only to steal and kill and destroy; I have come that they may have life, and have it to the full.

John 15:7

⁷If you remain in me and my words remain in you, ask whatever you wish, and it will be given you.

Acts 3:6-10

⁶Then Peter said, "Silver or gold I do not have, but what I have I give you. In the name of Jesus Christ of Nazareth, walk." ⁷Taking him by the right hand, he helped him up, and instantly the man's feet and ankles became strong. ⁸He jumped to his feet and began to walk. Then he went with them into the temple courts, walking and jumping, and praising God. ⁹When all the people saw him walking and praising God, ¹⁰they recognized him as the same man who used to sit begging at the temple gate called Beautiful, and they were filled with wonder and amazement at what had happened to him.

Acts 9:32-34

³²As Peter traveled about the country, he went to visit the saints in Lydda. ³³There he found a man named Aeneas, a paralytic who had been bedridden for eight years. ³⁴"Aeneas," Peter said to him, "Jesus Christ heals you. Get up and take care of your mat." Immediately Aeneas got up.

Romans 8:11

¹¹And if the Spirit of him who raised Jesus from the dead is living in you, he who raised Christ from the dead will also give life to your mortal bodies through his Spirit, who lives in you.

2 Corinthians 10:3-5

³For though we live in the world, we do not wage war as the world does. ⁴The weapons we fight with are not the weapons of the world. On the contrary, they have divine power to demolish strongholds. ⁵We demolish arguments and every pretension that sets itself up against the knowledge of God, and we take captive every thought to make it obedient to Christ.

2 Corinthians 12:9

⁹But he said to me, "My grace is sufficient for you, for my power is made perfect in weakness." Therefore I will boast all the more gladly about my weaknesses, so that Christ's power may rest on me.

Ephesians 6:10-17

¹⁰Finally, be strong in the Lord and in his mighty power. ¹¹Put on the full armor of God so that you can take your stand against the devil's schemes. ¹²For our struggle is not against flesh and blood, but against the rulers, against the authorities, against the powers of this dark world and against the spiritual forces of evil in the heavenly realms. ¹³Therefore put on the full armor of God, so that when the day of evil comes, you may be able to stand your ground, and after you have done everything, to stand. ¹⁴Stand firm then, with the belt of truth buckled around your waist, with the breastplate of righteousness in place, ¹⁵and with your feet fitted with the readiness that comes from the gospel of peace. ¹⁶In addition to all this, take up the shield of faith, with which you can extinguish all the flaming

arrows of the evil one. [17]Take the helmet of salvation and the sword of the Spirit, which is the word of God.

Philippians 4:6-7

[6]Do not be anxious about anything, but in everything, by prayer and petition, with thanksgiving, present your requests to God. [7]And the peace of God, which transcends all understanding, will guard your hearts and your minds in Christ Jesus.

1 Thessalonians 5:23-24

[23]May God himself, the God of peace, sanctify you through and through. May your whole spirit, soul and body be kept blameless at the coming of our Lord Jesus Christ. [24]The one who calls you is faithful and he will do it.

2 Timothy 1:7

[7]For God did not give us a spirit of timidity, but a spirit of power, of love and of self-discipline.

Hebrews 10:23

[23]Let us hold unswervingly to the hope we profess, for he who promised is faithful.

Hebrews 10:35-36

[35]So do not throw away your confidence; it will be richly rewarded. [36]You need to persevere so that when you have done the will of God, you will receive what he has promised.

James 5:14-16

[14]Is any one of you sick? He should call the elders of the church to pray over him and anoint him with oil in the name of the Lord. [15]And the prayer offered in faith will make the sick person well; the Lord will raise him up. If he has sinned, he will be forgiven. [16]Therefore confess your sins to each other and pray for each other so that you may be healed. The prayer of a righteous man is powerful and effective.

1 Peter 2:24

[24]He himself bore our sins in his body on the tree, so that we might die to sins and live for righteousness; by his wounds you have been healed.

1 John 3:8

[8]He who does what is sinful is of the devil, because the devil has been sinning from the beginning. The reason the Son of God appeared was to destroy the devil's work.

1 John 5:14-15

[14]This is the confidence we have in approaching God: that if we ask anything according to his will, he hears us. [15]And if we know that he hears us—whatever we ask—we know that we have what we asked of him.

Revelation 12:11

[11]They overcame him
   by the blood of the Lamb
   and by the word of their testimony;

they did not love their lives so much
as to shrink from death.

6. *Get the best medical opinion possible.*

There are more than 450,000 doctors in the United States. Do not go to just anyone. Find the doctor who is renowned for his or her expertise in the area of your health issue. (If you can find a specialist who is also a Christian — even better!) Notice that you should seek the best "opinion," not the best "treatment." The doctor will undoubtedly want to run tests to more thoroughly diagnose your problem and to understand your situation better. After the tests are completed and the diagnosis has been reviewed, resist jumping into treatment immediately. Now is your time to ask questions. Ask ten or ask one hundred! Ask until you are reassured that you know exactly what is going on in your body and exactly what each possible method of treatment entails. Then you can prayerfully consider your treatment options and get *the Lord's opinion* on how to proceed. Remember that you are the boss of your health and your body. Do not be intimidated by white lab coats and stethoscopes. Do not delegate your treatment choices to anyone else.

7. *Get the best chiropractic care possible.*

We have already discussed the amazing healing benefits of chiropractic care. If you are not currently seeing a chiropractor, revisit those chapters and find a passionate doctor of chiropractic now.[62] It has never been so vital that

---

62   See the Referral Directory in the appendix. Most all of the chiropractic doctors listed there are Christians whom I know personally.

the healing your body wants to perform be free to flow through your spinal column and out into each part of your body. Empower your body to heal itself as God intended!

8. *Find an excellent nutritionist.*

Chances are that the medical care you will be receiving will be aggressive and have some negative impact on your body. That makes it even more important to feed your body constructive foods and food supplements during this time of treatment and recovery. A good nutritionist will give you a thorough, natural approach to battle your condition and your diet will provide your body with much-needed nutritional tools to promote healing.

9. *Start an age- and condition-appropriate exercise program.*

Now more than ever you need fresh air, sunshine, oxygen and physical activity. Exercise will strengthen your body, improve your stamina, increase oxygen levels (disease hates oxygen) and will help you maintain a great attitude.

10. *Visualize yourself well.*

Take time daily and frequently to visualize yourself healed and whole. If you have lung cancer, picture your diseased lungs becoming pink and healthy again. If you have a tumor, see it shrinking in your mind. If you have suffered from a heart attack, visualize your heart strong and vibrant. If you have blocked arteries, imagine them opening up and blood flowing freely through them.

You may be thinking, "This is silly," or, "I do not have time for that." You have nothing but time, especially if your health is leading down a frightening path. The power of visualization has been proven for athletes; why not put it to use for the healing of your body?

There is every reason to hope and expect healing as you partner with God.

I have personally walked with many of my patients through a dreaded diagnosis and on to full health and healing following the principles outlined above. You have immense control over whatever medical situation you are presently facing and there is every reason to hope and expect healing as you partner with God. Do not sit back and resort to "Hope Management" for your recovery, and certainly do not leave your healing to chance or put your health decisions into the hands of another person. God has provided the strength, faith and innate healing that you need – they are at your disposal as His child! Pray that He will heal you and do everything you can to make that healing a reality in your life.

Lord, you know exactly what health issue I am facing right now. I thank you that you promised to never leave me alone and that you are walking beside me every step of the way. I ask you to release healing in my life and body. Help me to make wise choices about the best form of treatment for my health problem. Surround me with other Christians who will pray for me and encourage me on this journey toward wholeness. I will listen for your still, small voice leading me to health and healing. Amen.

A Prescription for Healing
– In Review

- IT IS NEVER TOO LATE TO BEING MAKING CHOICES THAT WILL LEAD TO DIVINE HEALTH AND HEALING.

- IF YOU HAVE BEEN DIAGNOSED WITH A HEALTH CONDITION, THERE ARE TEN STEPS YOU SHOULD TAKE TO PURSUE HEALING:

  1. BELIEVE PSALM 112:6-8.

  2. SPEND TIME IN PRAYER.

  3. RALLY THE TROOPS.

  4. BE ANOINTED FOR HEALING.

  5. TAKE YOUR SPIRITUAL MEDICINE.

  6. GET THE BEST MEDICAL OPINION POSSIBLE.

  7. GET THE BEST CHIROPRACTIC CARE POSSIBLE.

  8. FIND AN EXCELLENT NUTRITIONIST.

  9. START AN APPROPRIATE EXERCISE PROGRAM.

  10. VISUALIZE YOURSELF WELL.

- YOU HAVE IMMENSE CONTROL OVER WHATEVER MEDICAL SITUATION YOU ARE PRESENTLY FACING AND THERE IS REASON TO HOPE AND EXPECT HEALING AS YOU PARTNER WITH GOD.

What medical situation are you currently facing? _____

_____

_____

_____

What was your current level of health prior to this diagnosis?

_____

_____

_____

_____

Agree right now that it is never too late to start taking better care of your body. Make the commitment to change and lead a healthier lifestyle. _____

_____

_____

_____

Are there any of the ten steps that you are already pursuing?

_____

_____

_____

_____

What new steps can you add to promote even more healing in your body?_____

_____

_____

_____

Notes: _____

_____

_____

_____

_____

_____

_____

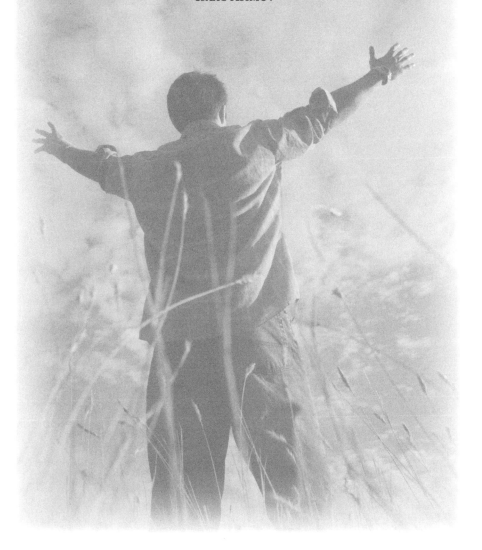

Life is pleasant. Death is peaceful.
It's the transition that's troublesome.

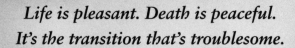

ISAAC ASIMOV

Chapter Twenty-Four

How Should a Christian Expect To Die?

YOU WILL PROBABLY NEVER BE INVITED to attend a Bible study entitled: "How Christians Should Die." This is kind of a shame, considering that each one of us will eventually face death — unless we are the blessed generation of saints who will be caught up with Jesus in the clouds when the Lord raptures His people.

Scripture says that the death of God's saints is precious in His sight.[63] He is not taken by surprise when one of His children slips into eternity, but guides their journey all the way home. In addition, we know that just before Stephen was stoned to death he saw heaven open and viewed Jesus standing

---

63   "Precious in the sight of the Lord is the death of His saints." Psalm 116:15

at the right hand of the Father.[64] What a glorious way to enter paradise!

God's will for you is to live a full, productive and victorious life, and then on the day that He has ordained you can die in a relaxed, peace-filled manner. It is my belief that if you have the "mind of Christ" and live each day sensitive to the leading of the Holy Spirit, you will sense when your time is at hand and you will be prepared and ready to meet your Savior.

> *God's will for you is to live a full, productive and victorious life.*

My oldest patient, Monte Stover, was 103 years old when he died. He enjoyed good health for his whole life except for his last month. He lived a long, productive life and drove his car until he was 97 years old. Monte was employed by Milton Hershey, the chocolate magnate. He went about lecturing about the history of our quaint picturesque town, Hershey, PA ("The Sweetest Place on Earth!"), until he was well beyond 100 years old. He credited daily exercise for helping him to live so long and well.

My next oldest patient, Martha Markey, was 96 years old when she died. She outlived several of her doctors and two of her three children. Martha was of sound mind and body up until three weeks before she died. She never experienced any pain as her body just slowly stopped working and she died at home in her sleep. Martha was not a health nut, but she did

---

64   "But Stephen, full of the Holy Spirit, looked up to heaven and saw the glory of God, and Jesus standing at the right hand of God. 'Look,' he said, 'I see heaven open and the Son of Man standing at the right hand of God.'" Acts 7:55-56

receive regular chiropractic care twice monthly for more than 60 years.

My great aunt, Trudy Weaver, died at the ripe old age of 95. Married to an old time osteopath, she believed in manipulation of the spine and received chiropractic care regularly for most of her adult life. Trudy lived a full, God-fearing and vibrant life and was healthy up until her last few weeks. Her passing was also both peaceful and painless.

Tragically, the long vibrant lives and relatively simple deaths I have just shared with you are not how most people walk into eternity. A good friend of mine just discovered how horrible a death from cancer can be as she cared for her father-in-law in her home. Bob had enjoyed a life relatively free from illness when at the age of 65 he started experiencing pain throughout his body. As his undiagnosed pain increased, a couple of over-the-counter pain medications a day turned into more and more until he was exceeding the recommended dosage in numbers that concerned the whole family. Doctors suspected arthritis and prescribed even more medication that simply did not alleviate his growing discomfort. Four months later, a bone scan finally revealed the culprit: lung cancer that had metastasized (spread) to his bones. The "hot spots" revealed on the scan were too numerous to count and the cancer had spread so far that the prognosis was two to three months. In two weeks' time, Bob was sleeping in a hospital bed, attached to an oxygen machine and only able to shuffle slowly from room to room because walking was so painful. Days later he was confined to a wheelchair. As his liver shut down, Bob's extremities swelled and his skin started leaking the fluids that his liver was unable to process. While his body shut down organ by organ, family members visited and tried to squeeze years of love and memories into his quickly fading days. *Five weeks after his diagnosis with stage four lung cancer, Bob died a very difficult and painful death.*

> *Christians who are walking in divine health can joyfully anticipate a healthy, vibrant life followed by a peaceful death in their old age.*

I am not suggesting that every person who succumbs to disease will die in such a horrible manner, or that every healthy person is immune to tragic circumstances. I do strongly believe, however, that Bob's death *is not* the way God intends for anyone to die. Christians who are walking in divine health can joyfully anticipate a healthy, vibrant life followed by a peaceful death in their old age.

Unfortunately, the majority of Americans rely on what I call "Hope Management." They hear of a friend or neighbor's diagnosis of cancer or multiple sclerosis and say, "Gee, I *hope* that never happens to me!" They continue making the same poor choices in eating and lifestyle and simply *hope* that disease stays far from their door. Then when a dreaded diagnosis is made, they devour every drug and aggressive treatment the medical establishment can offer, desperate for answers, continuing to *hope* for a cure. It is so much easier to stay healthy than it is to get healthy once you are diagnosed with a disease.

We do not have to live this way! I am here to tell you that *diseases don't just jump out of the blue and attack bodies.* Diseases show up where they are welcome. I understand that no one ever wished for a disease and that is not what I am suggesting. But sickness and disease occur for a reason. There is *always* a reason. Disease shows up because the tissue environment in a person's body is unhealthy and has hung out a "Diseases Welcome" sign. Just like flies gather on rotting garbage and fruit flies appear when fruit begins to go bad, disease finds an entry when health

> *Diseases don't just jump out of the blue and attack bodies. Diseases show up where they are welcome.*

is continuously compromised. If you clean up the garbage, flies won't appear, and if you maintain divine health, disease will be nonexistent as well. *Healthy bodies don't get sick; unhealthy bodies do.*

Your body is engineered to walk in divine health. Both sickness and health are consequences of our personal choices. Choices regarding what foods we eat, what thoughts consistently fill our minds, our level of physical activity, whether we keep our spine healthy, how we manage stress, how we deny or give in to our fleshly desires and the acceptance or rebellion of God's design for righteous living all accumulate. All of these choices produce either divine health and protection against disease or a welcome mat for one or more health disorders to take up residence.

Someone once said that if you do not want to be poor, do not do what poor people do. Conversely, if you want to be wealthy, copy what wealthy people do and you will eventually become wealthy, too. It is no different if improved health is your goal. Want to be healthier? Copy what you see healthy people doing, and do not mimic what you see unhealthy people doing. Do not want to be overweight? Do not eat what you see overweight people eating. Want to be fit and healthy? Find out what those people do and join them!

If you follow the strategies for divine health that I have laid out, I can all but guarantee you will greatly reduce the odds of ever receiving a dreaded diagnosis. Healthy people do not get diseases and they do not need a bunch of pills to cure them of those diseases. They make conscious choices to care for their bodies, souls and spirits, recognizing that they are partners with God in bringing His kingdom to earth and enjoying every day that He has ordained for them to live, laugh and love.

Father, thank you that I am not destined for disease and suffering but that you have enabled and empowered me to make wise choices. Help me to walk in divine health and keep sickness and disease far away from my life and my family. Thank you that I am not just a victim of whatever disease comes my way, but that you give me the strength to make wise choices to avoid them. Bless me as I joyfully live the exciting and productive days you have ordained for me. Amen.

How Should a Christian Expect to Die?
– In Review

- ☫ GOD'S WILL FOR YOU IS TO LIVE A FULL, PRODUCTIVE AND VICTORIOUS LIFE, AND THEN ON THE DAY THAT HE HAS ORDAINED YOU CAN DIE IN A RELAXED, PEACE-FILLED MANNER.

- ☫ THE MAJORITY OF AMERICANS RELY ON "HOPE MANAGEMENT." THEY HEAR OF A FRIEND OR NEIGHBOR'S DIAGNOSIS OF CANCER OR MULTIPLE SCLEROSIS AND SAY, "GEE, I *hope* THAT NEVER HAPPENS TO ME!"

- ☫ DISEASE SHOWS UP BECAUSE THE TISSUE ENVIRONMENT IN A PERSON'S BODY IS UNHEALTHY AND HAS HUNG OUT A "DISEASES WELCOME" SIGN.

- ☫ HEALTHY BODIES DON'T GET SICK; UNHEALTHY BODIES DO.

- ☫ WANT TO BE HEALTHIER? COPY WHAT YOU SEE HEALTHY PEOPLE DOING, AND DO NOT MIMIC WHAT YOU SEE UNHEALTHY PEOPLE DOING.

- ☫ CHRISTIANS WHO ARE WALKING IN DIVINE HEALTH CAN JOYFULLY ANTICIPATE A HEALTHY, VIBRANT LIFE FOLLOWED BY A PEACEFUL DEATH IN THEIR OLD AGE.

Have you had any loved ones die of "old age?" What was their death like? _____

_____

_____

_____

Have you watched anyone die of one of The Top Ten Killers? What did that process look like?_____

_____

_____

_____

Have you been relying on Hope Management? ("Gee, I *hope* that never happens to me!") _____

_____

_____

_____

Which seems simpler: to stay healthy and avoid disease or neglect your health and struggle to recover from disease?_____

_____

_____

_____

Have you inadvertently hung out a "Diseases Welcome" sign as a result of neglecting the proper care of your body? _____

_____

_____

_____

Think of the people you are modeling your life after. Is there anyone you are modeling your health habits after? Make the decision to start copying what the healthiest people in your life are doing. _____

_____

_____

_____

Notes: _____

_____

_____

_____

_____

_____

_____

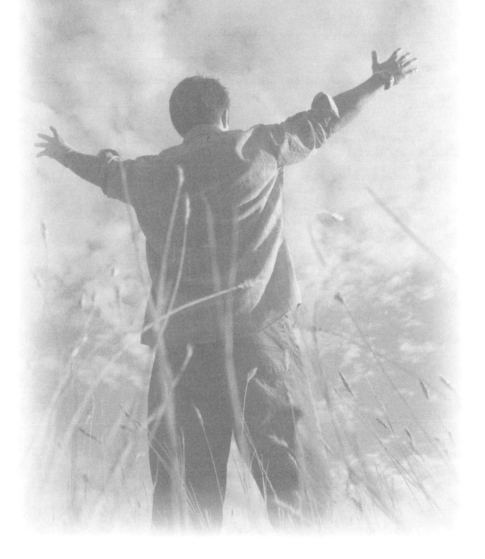

Have faith in God; God has faith in you.

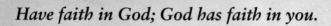

EDWIN LOUIS COLE

Chapter Twenty-Five

Becoming Fit for the King

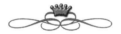

BECOMING "FIT FOR THE KING" is an exciting decision that all of heaven applauds. It lets God know that you are ready for service, waiting to be called into action in His kingdom and that you are capable of fulfilling every mission He gives you. God longs for all of His people to be prepared and eager to serve in the kingdom!

Because your body is constantly renewing itself through the replacement of cells, you become a "new you" about every 90 days. This is wonderful news, because it will only take three short months for you to have a body built on the strong foundation of good health!

You can think of your body as an automatic teller machine. Every time you make the choice to do something good for health (exercising, eating healthy

> *Becoming*
> *"Fit for the King"*
> *is an exciting*
> *decision.*

> *Every time you make the choice to do something good for health you are making a deposit in your health account.*

food, seeing your chiropractor, etc.) you are making a deposit in your health account. The more deposits you make, the healthier you will become. When you do get sick, there will be a balance available to withdraw from and you will quickly regain your health and physical wholeness.

If you are not sure where to start, following is a list of 11 simple steps we have discussed to become "Fit for the King."

1. *Recognize and be thankful that you are the crown of God's creation, wonderfully fashioned with an inborn ability to heal yourself. Treat your body with more care and respect than you would a priceless piece of art. Allow God's design for divine healing to fully function by taking good care of your body, mind and soul.*

2. *Soberly consider that God has pre-ordained your days. Make choices that will enable you to live to see them all and to accomplish all that He has planned for your life.*

3. *Take an honest assessment of your present level of health. Determine what changes you need to make to promote health and healing in your body and life.*

4. *Eat the healthiest, most constructive foods you can and avoid destructive foods.*

5. *Avoid toxins as much as possible. Maintain a healthy body that will be able to detoxify itself because you cannot completely avoid all toxin exposure.*

6. *Completely close the door on cancer and the other Top Ten Killers by following the strategies outlined.*

7. *Avoid prescription and over-the-counter medication whenever possible. Instead, rely on natural methods of healthcare for preventing and treating sickness and disease.*

8. *Limit stress in your life by careful prioritizing and intentionally scheduling your activities.*

9. *See a chiropractor for regular spinal care which will promote and enhance the innate healing ability God created in your body.*

10. *Increase your faith by meditating on God's word. Pray daily over yourself, your family and your possessions, pleading the blood of Jesus on your behalf.*

11. *When you do get sick, surround yourself with a group of strong Christians who will pray for your healing. Continue walking in faith, making decisions that will naturally strengthen your body.*

In Deuteronomy 30:19, Moses challenged the Israelites to make a monumental decision. "This day I call heaven and earth as witnesses against you that I have set before you life and death, blessings and curses. Now choose life, so that you and your children may live...." Following Christ has already brought eternal life to your spirit as a son or daughter of the King, but the same choice remains for your body. Will you make decisions that bring life or death to your body – the very temple that houses the Holy Spirit of the Almighty God? Do not be concerned if the choice seems overwhelming to you at first; just start making small changes and trust that God will continue to guide and direct you as you walk in greater levels of health. Those who walk in divine health never need a divine healing!

You have been wonderfully created, lovingly chosen and divinely commissioned to serve in God's kingdom. It is my fervent prayer that when God calls you into action on His behalf you will be ready and able to serve Him with all of your heart, soul and strength. Make wise choices, listen for His voice and be found "Fit for the King!"

Fit for the King Providers and Speakers Bureau

These Doctors Represent Some of the
Best Chiropractors in North America

ALABAMA

James Olszewski, D.C.
Wayne Stephens, D.C.
  Rocket City Chiropractic
  2417 Jordan Lane
  Huntsville, AL 35816
  ((256) 721-9696
  bigoski99@yahoo.com

ARIZONA

Mike Henriksen, D.C.
  Spinal Correction Center
  1327 E. Chandler Blvd Suite #106
  Phoenix, AZ 85048
  (480) 460-1177
  www.spinalcorrectioncenter.com
  turbo3d1@cox.net

CALIFORNIA

Phil Straw, D.C.
  Back Pain Relief Centers
  1810 Fullerton Ave., Suite 201
  Corona, CA 92880
  (951) 270-2883
  strawmanchiro@yahoo.com

CANADA

Michael Reid, D.C.
Lize Cloutier, D.C.
  Hampton Chiropractic & Wellness Centre
  1419 Carling Ave. Suite 209
  Ottawa, On. K1Z 7L6
  613-761-1600
  ottawawellnessnetwork@gmail.com

COLORADO

Daniel Knowles, D.C.
Richelle Knowles, D.C.
Network Family Wellness Center
1715 15th Street
Boulder, CO 80302
(303) 998-1000
www.networkwellnesscenters.com
frontdesk@networkwellnesscenters.com

Jeffrey Parham, D.C.
Wellness Rhythms Chiropractic
126 S. Madison Street, Suite C
Denver, CO 80209
(303) 722-1104
www.wellnessrhythmns.com
drparham@wellnessrhythms.com

Scott Hahn, D.C.
Leah Hahn, D.C.
Body In Balance Chiropractic, P.C.
710 Golden Ridge Road, #114
Golden, CO 80401
(303) 215-0390
www.bodyinbalancechiropractic.com
bibchiropractic@hotmail.com

DELAWARE

Jeanay Whye, D.C.
Abundant Life Chiropractic Center, LLC
5242 Summit Bridge Road
Middletown, DE 19709
(404) 993-5209
jeannay8@yahoo.com

FLORIDA

Christopher W. Hood, D.C.
E. Danielle Hood, D.C.
Erika Meister, D.C.
Hood Family Chiropractic Center
5590 54th Ave. N
St. Petersburg, FL 33709
(727) 544-9000
www.hoodchiropractic.com
info@hoodchiropractic.com

Jeffrey E. Raheb, D.C.
Raheb Family Chiropractic
6705 38th Ave. N., Suite B
St. Petersburg, FL 33710
(727) 381-3456
www.rahebchiropractic.com
Rahebchiro@yahoo.com

Michael J. Risoldi, D.C.
Risoldi Family Chiropractic
3023 Eastland Blvd., Bldg H101
Clearwater, FL 33761
(727) 797-9900
www.risoldi.com
drmike@risoldi.com

John Rauch, D.C.
Rauch Chiropractic Wellness Center
33385 US 19N
Palm Harbor, FL 34684
(727)-785-4830
rauchee2000@verizon.net

Cliff Zurkan, D.C.
Bay Area Chiropractic
10785 Ulmerton Road
Largo, FL 33778
(727) 518-1999
bacpainfree@aol.com

Rolando Toulon, D.C.
5560 S Flamingo Road
Cooper City, FL 33330
(954) 680-8182
rolandodc1@gmail.com

GEORGIA

Erin Arnold, D.C.
Amy Valente, D.C.
New Life Chiropractic
3451 Cobb Parkway NW #6
Acworth, GA 30101
(678)574-5678
drerinarnold@yahoo.com
dravalente@yahoo.com

O'Hara Moody-McKenna, D.C.
Aliyah Stotter, D.C.
Back 2 Back Chiropractic
1719-B Mount Vernon Road
Dunwoody, GA 30338
(770) 391-2771
info@back2backchiro.com

IDAHO

Amy Spoelstra, D.C.
15 W. Honeysuckle Avenue
Hayden, ID 83835
(208) 762-1414
dramy@spoelstrachiro.com

INDIANA

Brian McCarley, D.C.
  McCarley Chiropractic
  A Creating Wellness Center
  255 South 10th Street
  Noblesville, IN 46060
  (317) 565-1726
  www.mccarleychiropractic.com
  drbrian@mccarleychiropractic.com

KENTUCKY

Michael Leone, D.C.
Ellie Leone, D.C.
  Leone Chiropractic
  8131 U.S. Hwy 42, P.O. Box 215
  Florence, KY 41022
  (859) 371-3071
  chiroleone@yahoo.com

Michael Redman, D.C.
  Chiropractic Family Wellness
  7276 Burlington Pike
  Florence, KY 41042
  (859) 282-8006
  www.drmikeonline.com
  drredman@insightbb.com

LOUISIANA

Phil Smith, D.C.
  Smith Chiropractic
  525 E. New River St., Suite B
  Gonzales, LA 70737
  (225) 644-8671
  www.drphilfamilydc.com
  drphil@eatel.net

MASSACHUSETTS

Anthony Moncton, D.C.
  Westboro Spine & Holistic Health Center
  20 South Street
  Westboro, MA 01581
  (508) 366-6630
  www.westborospinehhc.com
  drmonton@westborospinehhc.com

Kevin Morey, D.C.
  Morey Family Chiropractic
  90 Main Street
  Leominster, MA 01453
  (978) 534-9500
  www.moreyfamilychiro.com
  drmorey@moreyfamilychiro.com

MARYLAND

James Roeder, D.C.
  Chiropractic Wellness Center of Baltimore
  8723 Belair Road
  Baltimore, MD 21236
  (410) 529-8010
  www.drroeder.com
  chirojamie@comcast.net

MICHIGAN

William Simpson, D.C.
Jennifer Simpson, D.C.
  Simpson Family Chiropractic
  3134 Fieldstone Drive
  Dexter, MI 48130
  (734) 424-0162
  drjennifer02@hotmail.com
  dr_w_simpson@yahoo.com

MISSOURI

Jason Harre, D.C.
  Harre Family Chiropractic
  869 St. Francois Street
  Florissant, MO 63031
  (314) 839-8884
  www.drjason.org
  drjason@swbell.net

Alex Vidan, D.C.
Sara Vidan, D.C.
  Vidan Family Chiropractic
  889 S. Brentwood Blvd., Suite 108
  Clayton, MO 63105
  (314) 678-9355
  www.drvidan.com
  dralex@drvidan.com

MISSISSIPPI

Eric Patten, D.C.
  Patten Family Chiropractic
  1227 Pass Road
  Gulfport, MS 39501
  (228) 863-7215
    www.pattenfamilychiropractic.com
    drpatten@pattenfamilychiropractic.com

NEBRASKA

Jason McCullough, D.C.
  Complete Health Chiropractic
  5640 South Street, Suite #3
  Lincoln, NE 68506
  (402) 488-0288
  completehealthdc@gmail.com

NEW JERSEY

Nicole Bonner, D.C.
  Healing Hands of Manahawkin
  230 Division Street
  Manahawkin, NJ 08050
  (609) 978-4304
  www.nicolebonner.com
  healinghandsofmanahawkin@yahoo.com

James Galgano, D.C.
Antonietta Galgano, D.C.
  Burlington Chiropractic
  321 West Broad Street
  Burlington, NJ 08016
  (609) 747-1100
  www.burlingtonchiro.com
  drjgalgano@yahoo.com
  ant8@hotmail.com

Keith Malinowki, D.C.
  Point Pleasant Chiropractic
  654 Ocean Road
  Point Pleasant, NJ 08742
  (917) 943-3859
  kword1@gmail.com

Tom Parkes, D.C.
  Bordentown Chiropractic Clinic
  231 Crosswicks Road, Suite 1A
  Bordentown, NJ 08505
  (609) 298-9820
  bchiro@gmail.com

NEW YORK

Randal R. Boivin, D.C.
  Upstate Chiropractic
  138 East Genesee Street
  Baldwinsville, NY 13027
  (315) 635-2333
  www.upstatechiro.com
  randyboivin@yahoo.com

Nathan Riddle, D.C.
  Riddle Chiropractic
  1183 Bay Road
  Webster, NY 14580
  (585) 670-0020
  www.riddlechiropractic.com
  nateriddle23@yahoo.com

Douglas Sullivan, D.C.
  B.C. Chiropractic
  3660 George F. Hwy
  Endwell, NY 13760
  (607) 754-5900
  www.bcchiropractic.com
  dcdougsully13@aol.com

Chad Wells, D.C.
Leah Wells, D.C
  Wells Family Chiropractic, PLLC
  1116 State Route 434
  Owego, NY 13827
  (607) 687-8787
  www.wellsfamilychiropractic.com
  wellsfamilychiropractic@yahoo.com

NORTH CAROLINA

Kevin Davis, D.C.
  Magnolia Specific Chiropractic
  1209-A Magnolia Street
  Greensboro, NC 27401
  (336) 285-8573
  magnoliaspecificchiropractic@gmail.com

OHIO

Robert DeMaria, D.C.
  North Coast Chiropractic
  Drugless Health Care
  362 E. Bridge Street
  Elyria, OH 44035
  (440) 322-3418
  www.drbob4health.com
  druglesscare@aol.com
Matt Finke, D.C.
  Finke Family Chiropractic
  6929 Miami Avenue
  Madeira, OH 45243
  (513) 272-9200
  www.finkefamilychiropractic.com
  info@finkefamilychiropractic.com

Brian Morris, D.C.
Misty Morris, D.C.
    Morris Family Chiropractic
    1640 Mentor Avenue
    Painesville Township, OH 44077
    (440) 639-9171
    www.brianmorrisdc.com
    mistynbri@aol.com

PENNSYLVANIA

Andrew D'Alessandro
    Eagle Chiropractic at Glenmoore
    1404 Horseshoe Pike
    Glenmoore, PA 19343
    (610) 942-9990
    www.eaglechiropractic.net
    drdalessandro@hotmail.com

Andrew Gottlieb, D.C.
    Eagle Chiropractic
    60 N. Pottstown Pike, Tommey Bldg Ste. 3
    Uwchland, PA 19480
    (610) 458-7777
    www.eaglechiropracitc.net
    aegottlieb@hotmail.com

Jack Herd, D.C.
Brian T. Carver, D.C.
    Herd Chiropractic Clinic
    2704 Market Street
    Camp Hill, PA 17011
    (717) 737-1681
    www.herdclinic.com
    herdclinic@aol.com

Tom Horn, D.C.
    Chiropractic Wellness Center
    27811 Route 220
    Athens, PA 18810
    (570) 882-9009
    www.familydc.com
    familydc@stny.rr.com

Charisse J. Huston, D.C.
    Huston Family Chiropractic &
    Wellness Center
    6100 Jonestown Rd., Suite A
    Harrisburg, PA 17112
    (717) 541-9668
    www.drhuston.com
    doccjh@msn.com

Jeff Ludwick, D.C.
    Camp Hill Family Chiropractic
    3401 Hartzdale Dr., Suite 117
    Camp Hill, PA 17011
    (717) 761-8840
    www.drludwick.com
    jaludwick@hotmail.com

Scott Maclary, D.C.
Christine Maclary, D.C.
    Maclary Family Chiropractic, LLC
    402 South Broad Street
    Lititz, PA 17543
    (717) 625-2223
    www.maclarychiro.com
    maclarychiro@dejazzd.com

David Madeira, D.C.
Angela Madeira, D.C.
    Madeira Chiropractic Center
    114 Prince Street
    Harrisburg, PA 17109
    (717) 545-4545
    drdavemadeira@comcast.net

Julie Madeira Niedwick, D.C.
    Madeira Chiropractic
    2507 Gettysburg Road
    Camp Hill, PA 17011
    (717) 766-9700
    www.docjulie.com
    madeirachiropractic@hotmail.com

John Madeira, D.C.
Kelli Ross, D.C.
J.D. Haynes, D.C.
    Madeira Chiropractic
    158 W. Caracas Avenue
    Hershey, PA 17033
    (717) 533-6100
    www.DrMad.com
    MadChiro@comcast.net

Walt Pierce, D.C.
    Pierce Chiropractic & Wellness Center
    2901 Mt. Roayl Blvd.
    Glenshaw, PA 15116
    (412) 213-0864
    walt442005@yahoo.com

Jeremiah Schreiber, D.C.
    River of Life Chiropractic
    2104 Zimmerly Road
    Erie, PA 16509
    (814) 866-2277
    www.riveroflifechiropractic.com
    drjerdc@velocity.net

Donald R. Rocklage, D.C.
Eagle Chiropractic of Pottstown
2091 Pottstown Pike
Pottstown, PA 19465
(610) 469-0700
www.eaglechiropractic.net
drocklage@parkercc.edu

Benjamin M. Grisafi, D.C.
Grisafi Chiropractic
507 W. Germantown Pike
Norristown, PA 19403
(610) 275-3355
www.drgrisafi.net

David S. Parker, D.C.
Family Tree Chiropractic
904 Dawn Avenue
Ephrata,PA 17522
(717) 738-2555
familytreechiropractic@hotmail.com

Selina Sigafoose-Jackson, D.C.
Kevin Jackson, D.C.
Sigafoose & Jackson Chiropractic
2816 E. Market Street
York, PA 17402
(717) 757-5731
www.sigafoosejackson.com
sig-jack@hotmail.com

SOUTH CAROLINA

Mike Geran, D.C.
Foothills Chiropractic
111 Fairview Pointe Drive
Simpsonville, SC 29681
(864) 228-6500
www.foothillschiro-sc.com
foothillschiro@gmail.com

Andrew Jackson, D.C.
Jackson Family Chiropractic
1025 West Carolina Avenue
Hartsville, SC 29550
(843) 332-6151
www.jacksonfamilychiropractic.com
jacksonfamilychiro@hotmail.com

Steven R. Amodeo, D.C.
Amodeo Chiropractic Clinic
161 Hwy 73 E
Collierville, TN 38017
(901) 853-8270
www.amodeochiropracticclinic.com
stevenamodeo@yahoo.com

Michael Bibb, D.C.
Bibb Family Chiropractic
1740 N. Germantown Pkwy, Suite 5
Cordova, TN 38016
(901) 752-4300
drmbibb@gmail.com

TEXAS

Terry Smedstad, D.C.
Woodway Wellness Family Chiropractic
4801 Woodway 175 E
Houston, TX 77056
(713) 622-2225
drsmedstad@yahoo.com

VIRGINIA

Mark Aldridge, D.C.
Caroline Chiropractic
17470 Center Dr., Suite 4C
Ruther Glen, VA 22546
(804) 448-0887
www.carolinechiro.com
drmark@carolinechiro.com

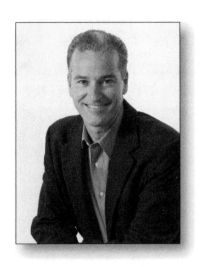

About the Author

DR. JOHN MADEIRA, one of the leading natural health and wellness experts, is pioneering the natural health and wellness revolution that is changing the face of health care and the way we look at sickness and disease.

Dr. Madeira graduated with cum laude honors from Palmer College of Chiropractic in Davenport, Iowa. He is in private practice and has personally cared for more than 20,000 of patients in his 30 year professional career. He lives in Hershey, PA with his wife, Karen and their two children.

John Madeira, D.C.
158 W. Caracas Avenue, Hershey, PA 17033

To sign up for his "free" email newsletter visit Dr. Madeira's website:
www.SettingThingsStraight.com

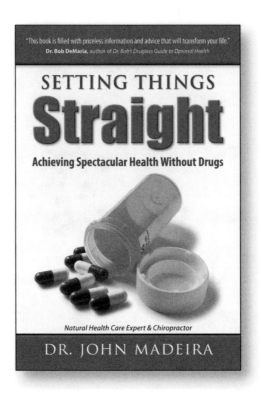

SETTING THINGS
Straight
Achieving Spectacular Health Without Drugs

Natural Health Care Expert & Chiropractor

DR. JOHN MADEIRA

"This book is filled with priceless information and advice that will transform your life."
Dr. Bob DeMaria, author of *Dr. Bob's Drugless Guide to Optimal Health*

Get ready to learn about a new and more natural approach to health care that focuses on fixing the root of the problem and not just treating symptoms with drugs. Dr. John Madeira *sets things straight* and reveals step by step how to enhance your body's ability to heal its self and achieve spectacular health naturally without drugs!

- ✓ Are you fed up with taking pills, dangerous side effects and exorbitant medical costs?
- ✓ Are you tired of how prescription drugs make you feel?
- ✓ Would you like natural solutions for your family's most pressing health issues?
- ✓ How much would it be worth to you to increase your energy, boost your immunity and lose weight naturally?
- ✓ Discover Dr. John's "million dollar" health habits and create your own Personal Wellness Plan!

TO ORDER: www.SettingThingsStraight.com
ISBN 978-1-60725-004-3

Public Appearances & Corporate Events

Dr. Madeira is available to speak at your Church, Christian Conference, Television or Radio Show, Corporate Event or Convention. His energetic speaking style will inspire, educate and motivate your church members, employees or network marketing downline to greater levels of health, fitness, personal confidence and motivation.

To schedule or inquire about an appearance, please contact Joyce Kapp at (877) 623-3472.

joyce@madeirasuccess.com
or visit www.SettingThingsStraight.com

MADEIRA SUCCESS STRATEGIES

(877)-623-3472

John Madeira, D.C.
Chiropractor, Success Coach, Author

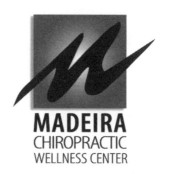

MADEIRA
CHIROPRACTIC
WELLNESS CENTER

To schedule an appointment at the
Madeira Chiropractic Wellness Center in Hershey, PA USA
Please call (717) 533-6100

Madeira Chiropractic Wellness Center (MCWC) is one of the busiest chiropractic practices in North America. With over 30 years of service to the community, the staff cares for nearly 1000 patients every week. MCWC's goal is to help families achieve and maintain optimal health through natural health care. The team is dedicated to educating the community about the many wonderful benefits of our drug-free and surgery-free method of health care.

Madeira Chiropractic Wellness Center
158 Caracas Avenue
Hershey, PA 17033
(717) 533-6100   www.DrMad.com

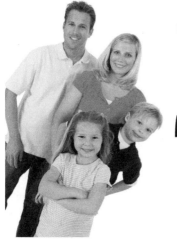

"A Healthy Spine Means A Healthier You!"

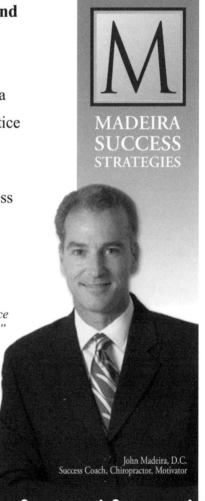